The
ULTIMATE
SEX TEST

Also by SMITH and DOE

What Men Don't Want Women to Know
The Book of Horrible Questions

The ULTIMATE SEX TEST

IS HE CHEATING? DOES HE LIE?

WHAT DOES HE WANT IN BED?

DARE TO TAKE THE TEST . . .

SMITH and DOE

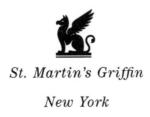

St. Martin's Griffin

New York

Library of Congress Cataloging-in-Publication Data

Smith, Mike.
      The ultimate sex test / Smith and Doe.
          p. cm.
      ISBN 0-312-25468-7
      1. Men—Sexual behavior. 2. Men—Psychology. 3. Man-
woman relationships. I. Doe, Bill. II. Title

  HQ28 .S557 2000
  306.7'082—dc21   00-023901

First St. Martin's Griffin Edition: June 2000

10 9 8 7 6 5 4 3 2 1

This book is dedicated to the

thousands of women who contacted us to

confirm our findings and

thank us for telling

the truth about men.

CONTENTS

FIRST, A WORD ABOUT SMITH AND DOE'S **ULTIMATE SEX TEST**

If you're reading this book, you're a woman who wants to know the truth about your man and his sexuality, no matter what the truth turns out to be. We congratulate you. You've made a wise choice. No general who plans for a great victory will enter the battle without learning everything he can about the basic nature of his enemy. By the same token, no woman who plans on a long and successful relationship should become involved with a man whose basic sexual nature remains a total mystery to her.

In this book we have expanded our previous revelations about the sexual appetites of men, their secrets and lies, into a foolproof set of formulas. For the first time anywhere, we provide *simple mathematical equations for arriving at the absolute truth about your man and his sexuality.* In *THE ULTIMATE SEX TEST* we quantify to a precise degree exactly what *your* man is capable of, and what he might be doing (or *wants* to be doing) at *any given moment.* If you are currently (or ever plan to be) in a relationship with a man, there's no getting around it— you *must* become a *student of male sexuality.*

Don't worry, you don't have to be Einstein to arrive at these mathematical solutions. If you can add, multiply, and subtract (or simply use a calculator) you will become a genius in the realm of your man's libido. Once you've got *that* nailed, you've got *him* nailed.

So, as *we* run for cover, put on your thinking cap, grab your calculator, sharpen your pencils, and get your man's number with **SMITH AND DOE'S ULTIMATE SEX TEST.**

HOW TO GO ABOUT SOLVING THE EQUATIONS

1. On a blank sheet of paper, *copy down the equation.*

2. Read each definition, then *fill in the correct number for each alphabetical factor.*

3. Perform the mathematical task for each set of factors *until you reach your conclusion.*

4. In "SCORING," *match your result* with the appropriate explanation.

The
ULTIMATE
SEX TEST

1

QUANTIFYING THE RELENTLESSNESS OF YOUR MAN'S *LIBIDO*

Once you have accepted the fact that **MAN IS A SEXUAL ANIMAL** who only remains faithful if he harbors a terrifyingly real fear of getting caught, you can begin to learn more about *your own man's* sexuality. Just how uncontrollable is your man's libido, you ask? Horribly, shockingly, revoltingly uncontrollable—*and that's if he's a priest*. Therefore, it is fitting that we begin with a formula that literally quantifies the miserable reality of *the relentlessness of your man's libido* (RL). Plug in the numbers and work out the following equation.

HOW SEXUAL AN ANIMAL IS YOUR MAN?

THE FORMULA

$$(AF) + (R) + (HF) \div (BP) = (RL)$$

THE VARIABLES

(AF) The first factor in this equation is your man's **AF** (Arousal Factor). If your man is easily aroused, chances are he's a true horndog. If it takes some effort to get his blood flowing, he's like a gun with the safety on (or recently *unloaded*). *As a* **SMITH AND DOE–Educated Woman** *you need to always keep in mind that the way your man acts with you is the reality of his sexual being. If he gets turned on when you wear a sundress, realize and accept that he gets turned on when he sees a random woman walking down the street in a sundress.* To determine his **AF,** *add up all the numbers that BEST DESCRIBE your man in the following hypothetical situations:*

He will get an *erection* if you . . .
Smile seductively at him. (**1**)

Accidentally brush against his crotch. (**2**)

Suggest something lewd. (**3**)

Blow in his ear. (**4**)

Bend down to pick up an onion from the kitchen floor. (**5**)

Come out of the john with a piece of toilet paper stuck to your shoe. (**10**)

(R) The horrifying overwhelmingness of your man's libido can also be judged by his **R** factor (what he would *rather* do than have sex). *Add up all the numbers that best describe your man.*

He would *rather* have sex than . . .
Eat. (**1**)

Watch a ball game. (**2**)

Make a big score in the stock market. (**3**)

Save a family in a fire and be hailed as a hero. (**4**)

Be able to lick his own balls. (**5**)

(**HF**) It's critical to quantify *how far* (**HF**) your man would go in order to have an orgasm. ***Once again, add up the numbers.***

With you out of town for a full year, he would have sex with . . .

Your best friend. (**1**)

Your sister or cousin. (**2**)

His secretary or direct underling at work. (**3**)

His secretary's mother. (**4**)

A duck. (**5**)

(**BP**) A true male sex-animal loses all brain power (**BP**) when aroused because the blood drains directly from his *big head* down to his *little head. Add up the numbers.*

When he is fully aroused, his IQ drops . . .

To room temperature. (**1**)

Maybe ten percent. (**2**)

Not at all. (**3**)

SCORING

$$(AF) + (R) + (HF) \div (BP) = (RL)$$

The *highest* and *most dangerous* score is (RL) = 50

$$[20 + 15 + 15 \div 1 = 50]$$

The *lowest* and *least dangerous* score is (RL) = 1

$$[1 + 1 + 1 \div 3 = 1]$$

If he scored 40–50, he's the ultimate sex beast. This is a man who is not only incapable of restraint but who, given the right circumstances, would pack your best friend, your sister, or even (if she's not a professional wrestler) your mother.

If he scored 30–40, he bears constant watching. It's okay to let him out of your sight as long as he's carrying a pager or cell phone, which is to say you should be able to detect his whereabouts at any given moment. Since men will probably not cheat if they fear getting caught, this is your bottom-line protection for a man in this category.

If he scored 20–30, you need to give him Viagra to get his libido going, but this is a good thing because he will only be turned on when you decide he should. Just to be safe, keep a count of his Viagra pills—if you notice one missing and unaccounted for, make him explain.

If he scored below 20, just call him *"NUMBNUTS."*

☺

Meditation for the Day

"A man who has no fear of me hearing his answering machine playback is a man who has no open affairs in progress."

♂

2

FORMULA TO DETERMINE YOUR MAN'S OFFICE FIDELITY FACTOR

In **WHAT MEN DON'T WANT WOMEN TO KNOW** we pointed out the fact that men, especially as they grow older, crave constant reminders that they are still attractive to women. *It is in the office that your man can truly cater to this need*, with the total security of knowing you will not interfere with or find out what he does when he is there. But now **SMITH AND DOE** have unearthed a magic formula that will, once and for all, tell you within a fraction of a percent how dangerously close he is to being unfaithful at the office. As we have said in the past, *if you ever saw the way your man behaves at the office you would become physically ill*.

In order to calculate your man's *Office Fidelity Factor* **(OF)**, you must begin with the assumption that **when he is with you** his mind is *95% free of unfaithful thoughts*. (*Even with the most well-intentioned man, you must always allow 5% for fantasies that* don't *include you.*)

THE FORMULA

$$95\% - (A\%) - (B\%) - (C\%) = (OF\%)$$

THE VARIABLES

(A) The single most critical factor in this equation corresponds to your man's position where he works. The higher he is in his company's hierarchy, the more his female coworkers will be sexually receptive to him. Unfortunately for you, this is a catch-22. If your man is a mailroom worker, he's relatively free from temptation. If your man is a CEO, the temptation never stops. The *horrible truth* is: If you're with a successful man you'd better hire a private detective and be afraid—be very afraid. But if you're "lucky" enough to be with a lazy, bankrupt slob, you've got nothing to worry about—*with regard to fidelity, that is.*

In order to determine **(A)**, select the ***one* number** that ***best describes*** your man:

Chairman of the board (**25**)
President, CEO, etc. (**20**)
Executive (**15**)
Mid-level worker (**10**)
Secretary, mail-room clerk, janitor, etc. (**5**)

(B) The next factor is the ***number*** of relatively attractive female coworkers your man encounters each day. (By "relatively" we mean free of humps, facial hair, or back hair). Include in your calculation ***only*** those women who are ***on the same (or lower) level of the company hierarchy*** as your man.

20 or more women (**20**)

10–19 women (**15**)

5–9 women (**10**)

1–5 women (**5**)

No women (**0**)

(**C**) Finally, you must factor in the ***type*** of women he works with. Pick a place from the list that ***best describes*** the general ambience of the women your man works with:

Miss America Contest (*real beauties*) (**5**)

Fashion Show (*dressing to please*) (**10**)

Blue-Collar Factory (*down to earth*) (**15**)

Chicken Coop (*talkers and flirters*) (**20**)

Pig Pen (*grateful for any attention at all*) (**25**)

Note: The numbers in this category appear inverted because most men stand a better chance of scoring office sex with an unattractive woman than a beautiful one.

SCORING

$$95\% - (A\%) - (B\%) - (C\%) = (OF\%)$$

A man's Office Fidelity Factor is lowest at 25%

$[95 - 25 - 20 - 25 = 25]$

His highest possible Office Fidelity Factor is 85%

$[95 - 5 - 0 - 5 = 85]$

If your man's Office Fidelity Factor is 25%: He's *definitely* involved with someone where he works at this very moment.

If his Office Fidelity Factor is 25%–35%: He's *probably* involved with someone where he works at this very moment.

If his Office Fidelity Factor is 35%–50%: He's sniffing around the workplace like a lost puppy to see which woman will show him any affection at all.

If his Office Fidelity Factor is 50%–75%: He's thought of having an affair with someone in particular, but he's decided she's too snobby for him and he doesn't want to be rejected.

If his Office Fidelity Factor is 75%–85%: He's so faithful to you he's probably even turned it down at the office (but that doesn't mean he'll hold off forever . . . .)

Meditation for the Day

"A man who hires another man as his assistant is concerned about work quality, not sex."

3

HOW TO DETERMINE WHETHER OR NOT YOUR MAN PRIVATELY FEELS THAT *Your Vagina* IS REVOLTING

One of the most common misconceptions by women is that their man, by virtue of his being with her, loves her vagina. Why else, they think, would the man stay?

The answer is this: Unless you had some form of sexual interaction the first night you met your man, by the time he saw the goods he was pretty much hooked. So even if he was relatively disgusted by what he found, he thought that it would A) grow on him or B) eventually get "repaired" by complaints he would lodge at a more comfortable time in the relationship.

*The reality is that your man **RIGHT AT THIS VERY MOMENT** may truly believe that your vagina is a stinky, hideous, revolting place that he only wants to visit in the dark of night when his brain cells are saturated with alcohol, praying that the encounter will end as soon as it began.*

So **SMITH AND DOE** have evolved this formula to allow you to learn the truth. And if you reach the unfortunate conclusion that your man does in fact believe that your vagina is revolting, you can at least confront him and hope to trim and scrub that stinking bush down to something more tolerable.

THE FORMULA

$$RF = H + ST + DL \times SF \div W$$

Revulsion Factor = Hair Content + Stench + Droopy Lips × Shower Factor ÷ Weight

THE VARIABLES

In order to accurately determine how your man feels about your vagina on a strictly physical basis, plug in the following variables, run the formula, and brace yourself for the results.

(H) Hair Content: This is a very important factor in determining whether or not your man secretly wants to don an outbreak hazard suit everytime you remove your undies. Why so important, you ask? Like an African jungle, the denser the forest, the more likely it is inhabited by countless forms of plant, animal, and bacterial life.

This variable should be *a number from 1 to 10*, **1** being *hairless* and **10** being *neanderthal.*

(ST) Stench: This variable, unfortunately, is one that you either have or you don't. Few people have ever "acquired" stench. It's like being born with a wandering eye: You can still function, but you don't want it. Another problem with this variable is that few women know how horribly their vagina actually reeks. *If you lined up every woman in the world whose vagina smells like a rotting wolverine corpse is lodged inside it and asked them, "How do you think your vagina smells?" not a single one will answer, "As a matter of fact, it's horrible. I wouldn't wish that stench on my worst enemy!"* Unfortunately for men, this is reality: Men usually have to find out how revolting the smell is firsthand, a discovery that is not unlike walking into a four-day-old multiple-homicide crime scene. So, in an effort to accurately determine the value of this variable, we ask you to stick your finger into your vagina. Then, making sure you aren't standing near any sharp objects (in the event of fainting), move the finger close enough to your nose to get a good solid whiff. Inhale.

The value of this variable is also on a scale of **1–10, 1** being the best smell and **10** being the worst. So, if your finger smelled like a flower, put a **1** here; if it smelled like a small possum infected with the black death crawled up there two weeks ago, put a **10** here. And for God's sake, be honest!

(DL) Droopy Lips: For reasons known only to God, there is a direct correlation between the size of a woman's vaginal lips and the stench emanating from her vagina. So take one more gander down there (if you put a **10** in the previous variable you can skip this section and head right to the showers) and tell us what you see.

If you can't see the lips from where you stand, they are probably small enough to warrant a **1.** If you can't tell whether you're looking at your vagina lips or your ankles, put a **10.**

(SF) Shower Factor: Good, consistent, and thorough cleansing of the vagina will make for a much more pleasurable experience for your man, regardless of what you found your Stench Factor to be. But few things are worse than a woman who doesn't take care of her vagina, properly cleaning it like a gun lover would clean his antique weapon or a car collector would polish his Ferrari. The cleaning of the vagina is imperative if you want to achieve a good score on this exam. So answer honestly.

On a scale of **1–10, 1** being thorough and consistent cleaning, with soap, at least twice a day, and **10** being a backpacker who likes to go on three jogs a day with no shower, plug in the number.

(W) Weight: As if fat people didn't have enough problems. Well, here's one more: If you're fat, your vagina is far more likely to smell like four-day-old feces.

This one's on a scale of **10–1, 10** being petite and **1** being a fat steaming monster.

SCORING

If you scored under 25: YOUR VAGINA SMELLS LIKE A FLOWER ON A SPRING DAY. Delightful to smell, taste, and touch, you are gifted and should be praised for your attention to detail and your understanding of the importance of a stenchless box. Your man is happy, and will be much less likely to stray knowing that he can't do much better—and if he tries, the one after yours will probably reek to the max.

If you scored under 150: YOUR VAGINA SMELLS OK. Sometimes it smells better than others. If your man attacks you right after a shower, he'll think he's died and gone to heaven. After a workout, it's smelling-salts time. You need to pay attention and make sure you keep that thing clean, or your man is going to be searching for streetwalkers just for the proverbial breath of fresh air.

If you scored over 150: YOUR VAGINA IS ACTUALLY ROTTING AS WE SPEAK. In all seriousness, your man fears close contact with your vagina like most men fear getting mugged and anally raped at gunpoint by the winner of the "Big Crane Convention" in Alabama. You need to begin the vaginal equivalent of HIV cocktail drugs. One of those bug foggers, followed by a hearty dose of Summer's Eve washed down with a gallon of ammonia. And that's <u>after</u> you shower.

Meditation for the Day

"The only reason (YOUR MAN'S NAME) *is with me is because at this moment in time he genuinely believes he can't do any better than me."*

4

FORMULA TO DETERMINE YOUR MAN'S POTENTIAL FOR ENGAGING PROSTITUTES

Prostitution exists.

And the only reason something exists is because there is a demand for it. You may want to think the demand for prostitutes comes from every man but yours, but that is like thinking the demand for food comes from everybody but you. Show us a man who has *never* been with a prostitute and we'll show you a man who has gone beyond college experimentation with homosexuality or has severe sexual dysfunction. You may ask why a man prefers a potentially skanky, disease-ridden *ho* to a loving girlfriend, mistress, or wife, but you may as well ask why the sky is blue. It *is* and he *does*. The answer to the first question, however, can be broken down into three parts: *no commitment, profound newness, and no guilt.*

No Commitment: Because a man considers casual sex no different from eating a hamburger, the ultimate sexual encounter (aside from you) contains no commitment whatsoever. A man makes no commitment when he buys a hamburger at McDonald's. He pays, eats, and leaves. Whether you like it or not, that is how men will take their sex whenever possible.

Profound Newness: It is programmed into the genes of all men, regardless of what they may say, to crave sexual variety. If it were the law of the land for a man to have either one wife or a harem, which do you think he would choose? Duh.

No Guilt: Because he has paid for the service, effectively buying off any emotional attachment from that particular sexual partner, he not only has no guilt, but feels proud of himself—as if, to spare your feelings, he went to McDonald's secretly because you are a vegetarian.

You can't stop your man from seeing a prostitute if that's what he is bound and determined to do. But with the following formula from **SMITH AND DOE**, you can ascertain how likely your man is to seek such sexual contact in the first place. Knowing how likely he is to seek out a prostitute gives you that all-important step up on cutting him off at the pass.

THE FORMULA

$$(NC \times 1) + (PN \times 2) + (DG \times 3) = (PP)$$

Note: Each factor is multiplied in order of its relative importance.

THE VARIABLES

(NC) No Commitment: This element measures his overall feelings about committing to relationships in general.

Select the number *that best describes* his attitude toward commitment in relationships:
"The worst torture on earth could not make me cheat on my woman." (1)

"I want my woman to know where I am every moment of
every day." (**2**)

"I would give a year's income rather than hurt my woman's
feelings." (**3**)

"I love being married." (**4**)

"I can make it on my own." (**5**)

"I love my wife, but what time do you get off work?" (**6**)

"Behind every great man is a great sexy mistress." (**7**)

(**PN**) **Profound Newness:** This factor gives you an idea of
his overall attitude toward ***newness versus oldness*** in the
various elements of his life. Select ***one number*** from each of
the following three sections, ***add them together,*** then ***multiply them by two*** to determine your man's (**PN**).

A. He gets a new car every . . .
10 years or more (**1**)

5 years (**2**)

3 years (**3**)

2 years (**4**)

year (**5**)

six months or less (**10**)

B. He changes residences . . .
Every 10 or more years (**1**)

Every 5–10 years (**2**)

Every 1–5 years (**4**)

Yearly or less (**5**)

C. He has been married . . .
Once (**1**)

Twice (**2**)

Three times (**3**)

Four times (**4**)

More than four times (**5**)
Never (**10**)

(DG) Degree of Guilt: The most important measure of your man's desire for prostitutes is how deeply he feels guilt where you are concerned. Select the statement *he would make that best describes* his level of guilt in his relationship with you:

"I feel guilty when . . ."
I like a movie and she doesn't (**1**)
I have fun at a party and she doesn't (**2**)
She wants me to work around the house and I don't (**3**)
I flirt with another woman in her presence (**4**)
I flirt with another woman when she is not there (**5**)
Another woman seduces me (**10**)
None of the above (**10**)

SCORING

$$(NC \times 1) + (PN \times 2) + (DG \times 3) = (PP)$$

He is *most likely* to see a prostitute if (PP) = 87
$$[7 + (10+5+10 \times 2) + (10 \times 3) = 87]$$

He is *least likely* to see a prostitute if (PP) = 10
$$[1 + (1+1+1 \times 2) + (1 \times 3) = 10]$$

If he scored 80–87 he may be with a prostitute at this very moment. This guy lies in bed at night thinking of prostitutes while you're playing with his hair.

If he scored 60–80 he's been with a prostitute within the last six months. And regardless of what he says or you may believe, six months before that, and six months before that, and so on, and so on, and so on . . .

If he scored 40–60 he's been with a prostitute within the last year. But then again, so has every politician, executive, and truck driver in the country, so it's not like your guy's alone or anything.

If he scored 20–40 he's been with a prostitute at least once in his life. Welcome to the human race—so has every guy.

If he scored 0–20 he wouldn't know a prostitute from a soccer mom. The only reason we can find that your man hasn't been with a prostitute is because he was either the ten-year-old victim of a pedophile or because the guy's so poor he can barely afford to pay attention.

Meditation for the Day

"Any man who claims to be disgusted by prostitutes is a man who can lie to me with a straight face."

5

FORMULA FOR DETECTING YOUR MAN'S LIES ABOUT HIS SECRET SEX LIFE

A man will lie about anything and everything to keep his sex life secret—from you, his friends, the world. No man on earth, including Howard Stern, will confess to everything he does in the shadows of his own privacy. What man wants the world to know he shoves his wife's vibrator up his own ass on a regular basis? Or that he secretly gets off on magazines like **Buck Naked Blubber Babes** and **Shitten Sie on Mein Face, Mein Herr!** or children's books like **The Little Sphincter That Could.** What man wants his best friend to know he fantasizes about fucking the best friend's wife? Or that he actually *is* fucking her? What man wants his wife or girlfriend to know that he makes his male secretary wear crotchless jockey shorts?

Like you, men are highly secretive about anything that could possibly embarrass them. As a result of this code of silence, we feel it necessary to arm you with a series of equations that will break down his lies in a variety of sexual areas. We begin with:

LYING ABOUT HIS LAST UNLOADING

CALCULATING HOW LONG IT HAS BEEN SINCE HE LAST UNLOADED

This is one of the most critical battles to be fought in the war to unearth your man's sexual secrets. Why is it so critical to know how long it has been since his last unloading? First, and obviously, if it differs in any way from *your* carefully recorded dates and times, it wasn't with you. If it wasn't with you there are only three possibilities: first, that it was some form of wet dream (proof of which must be found on his sleeping garments); second, that it was with someone else; and third, that it was a masturbatory episode (**See: "Non-Stick Equations to Determine the Frequency of Your Man's Masturbation"**).

Doctors (who are not afraid to speak out) recommend that you perform the measurements in this equation *on a random basis*, as with drug testing. This is the most efficient way to instill fear in your man and, as we now know, fear is the only thing that keeps him from unloading with anyone else but you.

THE FORMULA

$$(AE) + (VE) + (TNE) = (TESLU) \; (pronounced$$
$$TEZ\text{-}loo)$$

Note: (TESLU = Time Expired Since Last Unloading)

THE VARIABLES

(AE) Arc of Ejaculation. This critical factor has been too long overlooked by purported "experts" in the field of Loading & Unloading. Many years ago, before big-name medical journals were afraid to tackle a man's *arc of ejaculation* for the sake of political correctness, it was a common procedure for health professionals and wives to measure a man's sperm-throw (arc of ejaculation) in order to calculate the passage of time since his last ejaculation. The more time that passes after an unloading, the more sperm buildup takes place and the more a man's ejaculatory muscles loosen in anticipation of a greater contraction. (*Contraction pressure of the ejaculatory musculature is approximately the same in all men, regardless of weight or penis size.*) When the ejaculatory musculature contracts, we get the *arc of ejaculation*. The longer the sperm-throw, the more time elapsed since his last unloading.

To determine his *arc of ejaculation*, you must either have him masturbate in your presence or, if this unduly embarrasses him, masturbate him yourself on any surface that lends itself to measurement, such as a long-jump sand pit (with requisite markers) or an eight-foot-long glass coffee table. Carefully measure the distance between the tip of his penis and the farthest white splotch.

My man's arc of ejaculation measured out at . . .
Less than 1 inch **(1)**
More than 1 but less than 2 inches **(2)**
More than 2 but less than 6 inches **(4)**
More than 6 inches but less than 1 foot **(6)**
More than one foot **(10)**

(VE) Volume of Ejaculation. Obviously, the greater his volume of ejaculation, the more it has been building since

his last unloading. Measuring the volume of your man's ejaculation is a sticky prospect at best. It is best to use a shallow
container, like a baking or casserole dish. Keep in mind that
his ejaculation must be full and complete in order for you to
obtain a precise measurement of the volume. Most men
require a minimum of three to five minutes of concentrated
post-ejaculatory milking (**CPEM**, in clinical terms) in order
for you to be sure that they are fully and completely unloaded. Once you have gotten every last milliliter of sperm
into the container, use a measuring spoon to collect the fluid.
This is the only correct, proper, and medically sanctioned
way to measure the true volume of a man's ejaculation.

The volume of my man's ejaculation is equal to . . .

¼ tablespoon **(1)**

½ tablespoon **(2)**

1 tablespoon **(4)**

1¼ tablespoons **(8)**

1½ or more tablespoons **(10)**

(TNE) Time Needed for Ejaculation. This is the easiest
factor of the three to arrive at. Using an ordinary stopwatch,
begin timing from the moment of full erection. If you are not
sure exactly *when* full erection began, check the vein which
runs just under the skin along the top of the penis shaft*. (No,
not the ulcerated lesion, the vein.) If said vein appears fully
engorged and blue in hue, the penis is in full erection. Con-
tinue timing until masturbation leads to ejaculation. End tim-

*If the erection was there before you started, he may be a victim
of DEADLY SPERM BUILDUP (DSP) and must be unloaded
immediately for medical reasons. Either that or he just came
home from packing your sister.

ing at the first emergence of white fluid, regardless of its con-
sistency. This is the *time needed for ejaculation.* If it takes
thirty seconds or less for him to ejaculate, your man has not
unloaded for some time. If it takes five minutes or longer, he
may well have ejaculated within the last several hours.

It took my man _____ to ejaculate.
thirty seconds (**10**)
one minute (**8**)
more than one but less than three minutes (**4**)
more than three but less than five minutes (**2**)
more than five minutes (**1**)

SCORING

(AE) + (VE) + (TNE) = (TESLU)

Period of time since last unloading is *longest* at 30.
[10 + 10 + 10 = 30]

Period of time since last unloading is *shortest* at 3.
[1 + 1 + 1 = 3]

**If your man scored 3–6 you may consider him a scurvy,
lying sack of shit for even wasting your five minutes by
not copping to fucking around in the first place,** not to
mention the fact that he *is* fucking around, for all you know
with an AIDS-ridden sixteen-year-old jailbait Haitian hooker.
DUMP THIS MAN BEFORE HE STARTS *FAKING ORGASMS*
when he's inside you.

**If your man scored 7–15, he's probably been beating off
in a highly irregular pattern in order to mix up your**

measurements. MAKE THIS MAN STAND WITH HIS PANTS AT HIS KNEES AND MASTURBATE ONCE MORE FOR PROOF OF FIDELITY.

If your man scored 16–24 he's the kind of guy who could knock out a charging bull with his force of ejaculation. If he in any conceivable way fits this description it is suggested you wear a protective helmet while conducting the test. THIS MAN'S EXUBERANCE IS INFECTIOUS: GIVE HIM TEN MINUTES TO RELOAD AND EXPOSE YOUR TARGET.

If your man scored 25–30, congratulations! Get a large rectangle of black velvet and *keep him spritzing on it*—you may have the new millennium's Jackson Pollock on your hands (pun intended).

☺

Meditation for the Day

"A man who lies about his past is lying about his present."

6

FORMULA TO DETERMINE YOUR MAN'S PREDILECTION TO ENGAGE IN THE AGE-OLD CONSPIRACY OF **MEN HELPING MEN**

Men, members of a secret fraternity from the day they draw their first breath, always help other men. Whether by lying, cheating, stealing, or any number of other underhanded techniques, a man will always help another man pull the wool over a woman's eyes, even if those two men have just met minutes before. Keeping this in mind, realize that *ANYTIME A MAN HAS TOLD YOU SOMETHING ABOUT YOUR MATE THAT WAS UNSOLICITED, NOT ONLY SHOULD YOU REGARD IT AS A LIE, BUT BELIEVE THAT THE EXACT OPPOSITE IS TRUE.*

Now that you realize everything you believed about your

mate until this point is a flat-out lie, you can begin the heal-
ing process by using the formula below as a way to help you
understand just how bad the damage is.

THE FORMULA

$$(P) + (NR) + (AP) \div (ON) = (HLIAL)$$
Note: (HLIAL = His Life Is A Lie)

Your man's friends have no doubt been kind enough to
inform you that your man has been such a good guy in his
past, he's never even touched a prostitute like all the other
guys in the group *(a common ploy—the good of the one out-
weighs the good of the many, who in this case don't care
because they're not depending on their friend's girlfriend
for sex anyway).*

So the questions we're about to ask you are about **HIS
FRIENDS**. *Because whatever your man says about
his friends is actually the truth about him, and
what you are witnessing is yet another SMITH AND
DOE– FOILED ATTEMPT to pull the wool over your
eyes.*

THE VARIABLES

The first variable, **(P)**, is meant not as a criticism of the use
of prostitutes, but as an indicator of your man's ability to
turn off his emotions and engage in sexual relations with
a nameless, disease-ridden stranger while paying for the
privilege.

When you asked your man if "his friends" use prostitutes, he said:

He assumes so. (1)

They've been with a few, but never had anything except oral sex. (2)

Yes, one of his friends has been with one, but she didn't charge him. (3)

They've never been with one, ever, how dare you even ask him that? (4)

He couldn't possibly count how many his friends have been with. (10)

The next variable we'll address is **NR (No Rub)**. This is an indicator of how many times your man has had sexual relations with nameless strangers without using condoms, a factor that affects you directly, as well as the insurance company when they wind up having to foot the bill for your HIV treatments.

When you ask your man whether or not "a certain friend" wears condoms during one-nighters with anonymous females, he says:

His friend wouldn't have sex until they were both tested for HIV. (1)

His friend had sex, but always wore a condom without complaint. (2)

His friend always wore a condom, but complained like hell. (3)

His friend has sex all the time without a condom. (4)

His friend has anal sex left and right without a condom. (10)

Speaking of anal sex, there's your man's **AP (Anal Past)**. There's nothing wrong with a man who loves anal sex, but just keep in mind that if he's done it with a lot of girls, he's susceptible to being tempted by a new one (the need for anal sex is a strong, erotic urge, and thus one of women's most potent siren songs), so you need to keep giving the goods or he'll get it elsewhere.

With regard to anal sex, your man's "friend":
Never had it, never had any interest in it. (1)
Always wants it, but his girlfriend never let him. (2)
Did it with his girlfriend, but says it was his first time. (3)
Does it a lot. (4)
Did it less than an hour ago. (5)

Finally, there's the mother lode of secrets, the secret that all men strive to protect each other from unveiling. The **ON (One-Nighter)** is a potentially devastating piece of mathematical info that can define your man's sexual character in an instant. Of course, if you ask his friends, he only fools around with girls he really likes or is in love with. **THIS IS A TOTAL CROCK OF SHIT.** Now that we've got that out on the table, ask him if his friends have a lot of one-nighters.

When you asked your man how many one-nighters "his friends" have, he said:
"They've had a few, but they didn't mean anything." (5)
"They've had a few, but usually didn't have sex
with them." (4)
"When they were younger they had their share, but after growing up, maturing, and realizing that empty one-night stands just left them feeling an intangible hollowness, they stopped having them. For a month." (3)
"Do you have a calculator handy?" (2)

[sweating] "They, I, I mean, they didn't do anything while you, I mean, his girlfriend was away! I swear! I mean *he* swears!" (1)

"What's a one-nighter?" (0.5)

SCORING

The highest achievable score is HLIAL = 50. *If your man scored near this number, you couldn't begin to imagine the amount of fungus that now calls your uterus home.* Your man can try to hide behind the human shields that are his friends, but you know the truth. This guy makes his worst friend look like a celibate monk.

If he scored between 30–40, *he's got a lot to hide, but he isn't hopeless.* Keep him on his toes at all times and realize what you are dealing with. You've got a guy who will not only do horrible things countless times, but he'll blame his best friends for it behind their backs!

If he scored between 20–30, *he's the typical man.* By women's standards, he's done some hideous things. By male standards, he's an average, good guy.

If he scored between 5–20, *he's a keeper.* This is a guy who is honest with you and doesn't need to hide behind his friends' lies. He has braved his way out of the fraternity of men to maintain an honest, trustworthy relationship with you. (*Who are we kidding? This entire paragraph is a men-helping-men ploy!*)

If he scored under 5, *SMITH AND DOE are concerned that your man could possibly be a "mo,"* *chowing helmet and packing sphinct whenever the opportunity arises.* This man's idea of a great meal is four blowjobs followed up with a rectal Roto-Rooter. Beware!

☺

Meditation for the Day

"When I suspect (YOUR MAN'S NAME) *of a transgression, I can be 100% sure he is guilty if any other man comes to his defense unsolicited."*

7

HOW TO DETERMINE WHETHER OR NOT YOUR MAN IS GOING TO **MARRY** *YOU*

Before we begin, remember the **SMITH AND DOE** maxim that you should know by heart by now:

THE ONLY REASON YOUR MAN IS WITH YOU IS THAT, AT THIS VERY MOMENT, HE GENUINELY BELIEVES HE SIMPLY CAN'T DO ANY BETTER.

Once you've accepted this as truth, you can begin to understand why the mere fact that your man is with you by no means indicates he is planning on marrying you.

There are countless men who are with their women because it's the best thing they've got so far; *but*, they think, *who knows who I may meet in the future? She will probably blow away this girl I'm with now*, they think, *so why get married now?*

Rather than risk being the faithful girlfriend who winds up getting the boot three years later because something better,

younger, and with bigger breasts comes along, use this formula to find out his **LM**—Likelihood to Marry—now, before
it's too late.

THE FORMULA

$$LM = PR + BM + FS + FC + LD \times YFP \div P$$

THE VARIABLES

PR (Past Relationships): The type, length, and quality of
your man's past relationships are a crucial indicator of future
results. If your man has never had a long-term relationship
before yours and he's older than twenty-one, you have about
as much chance of getting married in the near future as we
have of getting pregnant.

    Score him on a scale of 1–10, 1 being a man who has
never had a long-term relationship and **10** being a man who
has had numerous fulfilling long-term relationships but just
"never found the right woman for marriage."

BM (Beliefs Regarding Marriage):
    Score him on a scale of 1–10, 1 being a man who
doesn't believe in the institution of marriage and **10** being a
guy who has been searching for the right woman and "can't
wait to get married."

FS (Financial Status): Believe it or not, your man's financial status is directly proportional to his desire to get married. The wealthier a man becomes, the more capable he
feels of providing a good life for a wife and, ultimately, kids.
A man with no money will use excuses to postpone marriage
because he feels financially inadequate. So, while you can

use this knowledge to address your man's specific situation (i.e., let him know that you don't care about money. Hold on, we're still laughing. OK, we're back.), you still need to plug in a number here.

Score him on a scale of 1–5, 1 being a guy who is poor and **5** being a guy who's rolling in it.

FC (Financial Controls): A man will not marry a woman unless he feels he can fully and completely trust her with his finances. That's not to say men will simply hand over access and controls; on the contrary, few men ever would be that foolish. But if he feels that you won't run around like an idiot on a spending spree if given a credit card, and that he can trust you to have access to some of his accounts if he needs you to do basic things like write a check or two or make a transfer, you'll be much closer to marriage.

Score him on a scale of 1–5, 1 being a guy who wouldn't let you touch his money if it meant saving his life and **5** being a guy who would trust you completely (and has shown evidence of this, not just your opinion).

LD (Length of Dating): The longer you've been with your man the more likely he is to believe deep inside that you are "the one."

So this variable is on a **1–10 scale, 1** being a year or less and **10** being ten years or more. You can figure out the in-between.

FP (Your Financial Problems): A woman burdened by financial problems of her own doing is a woman likely to cause her man financial problems as well. Whether or not this **SMITH AND DOE** adage is true is irrelevant—it's what your man will believe. So either keep your troubles secret or blame them on someone else.

Score this on a scale of 1–5, 1 being a financial disaster and **5** being perfect finances. Describe yourself using this variable.

P (Pressure): The amount of pressure you exert on your man to marry you is inversely proportional to the possibility of an actual marriage taking place. In other words, the more pressure, the less chance. Men don't respond well to this kind of pressure, so if you're thinking about giving an ultimatum anytime soon, think again—many relationships that might have ultimately resulted in marriage end prematurely as a result of pressure being applied where it shouldn't have been.

   Score this on a scale of 1–5, 5 being a lot of pressure and **1** being none. Plug in the number.

SCORING

If your man scored 150–200, you are definitely the love of his life and he is anxiously looking forward to the right opportunity to propose. You will live a long and fruitful life with this man, and as long as you don't read our first book, **WHAT MEN DON'T WANT WOMEN TO KNOW**, you'll be blissfully unaware of his constant infidelities.

If your man scored 100–150, you are Miss Right Now, and maybe you'll become Miss Right, but it isn't looking too good. This guy, while seemingly happy, is subconsciously waiting for the bigger, better deal to come along so he can jump off your tugboat and onto her speedboat. Thus, it is advisable that you be keeping a similar eyes-open attitude, because it could be a matter of minutes before you get the boot.

If your man scored 50–100, the only two things that are going to make him get married are if you're pregnant with twins and his dad's the pope, or if your father decides to have a conversation with him and his good pals Smith & Wesson.

If your man scored under 50, it's a miracle this guy returns your calls. Your man is probably with you solely for the ease of access to sex. So if you're enjoying the sex, great. If you're expecting a ring, go press the doorbell, because that's about as close as you're gonna get with this guy.

☺

Meditation for the Day

"Stare assieme é un eufemismo che sta per tenere una ragazza fuori dal mercato dal punto di vista sessnale. Il matrimonio non fa altro che rendere la cosa permanente."

TRANSLATION

"Dating is a euphemism for keeping a girl off the market sexually. Marriage merely makes this permanent."

8

FORMULA TO DETERMINE IF YOUR MAN HAS EVER *"EXPERIMENTED"* WITH HOMOSEXUALITY

"Experimented with homosexuality" is a nice way of describing such lovely acts as *plugging butt, chowing helmet, and picking up soap in the men's shower.* Outside of openly-declared gays, there isn't a man in the world who will admit to ever having been a *mo.* Now, it's entirely possible that you don't want to know if your man has ever engaged in these activities, but **SMITH AND DOE** are here to tell you that you'd better find out. Why? Because statistics tell us that 85% of all men who "experimented" at some stage of their life will do it again in the future, even if they are in a committed relationship with a woman. This occasional "experiment" will eventually become a full-fledged clinical trial, requiring daily research for years to come.

This revelation is not merely a scare tactic dredged up to make this book indispensable to women. It appears that, like hepatitis or herpes, **DLHB (Disproportionate Love of**

Hairy Butts) is an affliction that remains in a man's system all his life. Even if it never gets physically triggered again (thus remaining dormant in the cells until prompted by some irresistible, hairy, sweaty beast of a man), the possibility that it might will always hang over your head like a sword of Damocles (*the famous Greek poofter*).

The trick is to know *if* your man "experimented" with homosexuality, and to apply your knowledge to keep him from backing into it again. To that end, there are two important equations for you to work out.

THE FORMULA

$$(GF) + (CC) + (TM) + (BF) + (GL) \times (AP) = (HE)$$

Note: (HE = His Homosexual "Experimentation" Factor)

THE VARIABLES

(GF) Gay Friends. Many women love to hang out with gay guys, shop for clothes and antiques, go to lunch, have drinks, and/or cry on their shoulders about their romantic woes. They feel safe, enjoying a special kinship with gay guys, as they both share similar sensibilities. Sometimes they even want sex with gay guys—not realizing that this fantasy always leads to a *dead end*. Gay guys choose **not** to mix with straight men except when absolutely necessary—primarily in business dealings, social engagements engendered by business dealings, or family imperatives. A straight man who has a large number of gay friends is at highest risk of contracting the dread *sphinctus rambunctus* (*the susceptibility to over-garrulousness of one's anus*). In case you're thinking this whole thing is about **SMITH AND DOE** waxing homophobic, *it's not*—although **SMITH** *does* exhibit that attitude *(he's in denial of his own homosexual tendencies and acts out to throw himself and everyone else off the track).* If your man already has several gay friends or, worse yet, suddenly starts introducing you to new gay guys because, "You'll love them!" or, "They're a hoot!" be warned—he's not completely "your" man anymore. And if he ain't only yours, you know whose he is—*birds of a feather pack together.* To determine **(GF),** *allow one point for each statement that is true for your man:*

Regarding my man's friends:
Some are gay but still in the closet.
Some are admittedly but quietly gay.
Some are Flaming Queens.
Not a single one of them is gay.
They would literally kill him if they found out he was gay.

(CC) Career choices. Men who have "experimented" with homosexuality have also "experimented" with careers like interior decoration, fashion design, and coal mining. "Coal mining?" you ask, eyebrows askance. Believe it or not, you'll find more homosexuals in a coal mine than a Broadway musical. A coal mine has the same irresistible combination of maleness, toughness, and darkness that makes most gay bars the treats they are. Any dark, crowded place where tough, sweaty, crusty men get together away from the scrutiny of women is a **DLHB** man's delight.

But if, for instance, your man is a big, bad, truck-driving teamster, the chances are much slimmer that he'll slip away to the other side (the *backside*, as it were). Unless, of course, he attends too many union meetings and comes home bearing the stains of some other guy's transmission fluid.

On the other side of the coin, if your man is a hard-driving

CEO of a big company, check back into his personal history to see if, for example, he did ironing and sewing to pay for business school. Or if he spent a spring break as a makeup intern at *Playgirl*. The careers your man chooses to plug away at parallel the holes he chooses to plug.

Score one point for each job skill your man possesses.
Sewing
Ironing
Baking
Decorating
Toe Dancing

(TM) Taste in Music. If your man insists on dragging you off to every Barbra Streisand concert, *wake up*. Is he playing a lot of Teddy Pendergrass around the house? Is there a Liberace poster in his top drawer? Does he hum Boy George in the shower? A man who cries to old Judy Garland records, whistles to Barry Manilow, and dances to the Village People needs to up his intake of heavy metal and gangsta rap. Music is an erotic stimulant! Believe it! When *you* want to hear The Rolling Stones' "Honky Tonk Woman" and *he* wants to play Bobby Short singing "Why Can't a Woman Be More Like a Man?" you can be assured the conflict in your musical tastes is a clear and present echo of the conflict in your erotic tastes. To determine his **(TM)** *score one point for each of the following types of music he enjoys*.

My man loves to listen to:
Andrew Lloyd Webber (Instrumentals)
RENT (Original Cast Album)

Bette Midler

Barbra Streisand

Kenny G.

Yanni

The Benedictine Monks

The Chipmunks

(BF) Bitchiness Factor. Sometimes, when a woman is in a bad mood, men call her *"a c—t."* **SMITH AND DOE** do not condone this demeaning behavior but merely call your attention to it. Often when a gay man is in a bad mood, other gay men call *him "a c—t."* All we are saying is, *"A c—t's a c—t,"* whether she's a woman or a *mo.* Guys who *don't* "experiment" with homosexuality don't get into random moods where their primary goal is to hideously humiliate, in ten-minute bursts, anyone who happens to cross their path. Guys who *do* "experiment" with homosexuality are capable of breaking out into sobs at any time of the day or night. If your guy is the *Wicked Witch of the West* one minute and *Camille* the next, you can bet he has done some serious "experimenting." The higher his **Bitchiness Factor,** the greater his chances of being found on Santa Monica Boulevard late at night wearing clam-diggers, "experimenting" with passing cars driven by men wearing bags over their heads. To determine your man's **(BF),** *score one point for each of the following statements that are true for him* (for a possible total of 5).

My man snipes at me whenever . . .

I don't do something exactly the way he wanted it.

He gets off the phone with his mother.

I wear mismatching accessories.

He gets a headache.

We shop for antiques.

(GL) Geographical Location. If he lives in San Francisco, the odds are 3:1 he's a *mo.* If he's in New York City, chances are that if he didn't actually "experiment" he's doing some *basic research.* On the other hand, if he's a Fairfield, Iowa man, chances are the only youthful "experimentation" he did was with livestock (and since he probably doesn't know whether the cow was male or female, thus freeing him from concerns of having packed a dude cow), and he is likely to consider himself normal. *Where* a guy lives says a lot about *how* he lives. Gay guys don't flock to Amarillo. Straight guys don't flock to Fire Island, grease up their bodies and wink at other men—with their sphincters. Big cities like Los Angeles, New York, and to a lesser degree Miami offer more possibilities to "experiment" with aberrant sexual behavior, if only because of the large population. It's easier for a man to get "lost" for an hour getting oral sex down on Mulberry Street or giving it on Hollywood Boulevard than to have a "secret" fling with the local blacksmith in the small town where he lives. (Not that some *small* communities aren't rife with *mos*— look at Disneyworld.) To determine your man's **(GL)** factor, *score one point each for the following:*

My man lives . . .
In a populous state.
In a populous city.
In a populous neighborhood.
In a neighborhood loaded with boutiques.
On a street where many other men walk dogs the size of cockapoos or smaller.
In a building where everyone looks like The Marlboro Man and lisps.

And last but not least . . .

(AP) Anal Preoccupation. This refers to certain of his physical tendencies *while engaging in sex with you.* If he acts like there is no such orifice as an *anus*, multiply the total of all previous factors by one (1). If he is preoccupied with *your* anus, multiply the equation by two (2). If he is preoccupied with *his* anus, multiply by five (5). If he is preoccupied with everything that reeks of *any rectal region whatsoever,* *multiply by ten (10).*

SCORING

$$(GF) + (CC) + (TM) + (BF) + (GL) \times (AP) = (HE)$$

Your man is *most* likely to have "experimented" with homosexuality if he scored 240 points.

He is *least* likely to have "experimented" with homosexuality if he scored 2 points.

If your man scored 220–240: Carefully mark the level on your lipstick. Chances are ten to one he's painting his lips when you're not around.

If he scored 200–220: Ground him immediately—no more "nights out with the *boys.*"

If he scored 180–200: Forget about the boys and the lipstick, but check his underwear for tell-tale signs of male visitors.

If he scored 150–180: You're edging toward safe territory. He may have "experimented," but with a little luck the results could have given him permanent homophobia (as in the case of **SMITH**).

If he scored 100–150: He's no more likely to have "experimented" than, say, a proctologist on a busman's holiday.

If he scored 50–100: When he sees a male anus wink its hairy eyelashes at him, he'll run in abject terror into your soft, loving arms.

If he scored 2–50: This guy is so straight that when he was a child, the doctor broke three rectal thermometers trying to take his temperature.

Meditation for the Day

"An unknown male 'friend' of (YOUR MAN'S NAME) *who suddenly needs* (YOUR MAN'S NAME'S) *emotional support is most likely, in reality, a woman."*

9

PERVERSITY
and Your Man

The most insidious danger that can threaten your relationship is *lack of sexual communication*. According to our research—over 1,100 anonymous interviews with men via the Internet—at least 90% of them harbor "depraved" sexual desires they will never communicate to their mates for fear of embarrassment and/or criticism *(but will eventually satisfy with someone else)*.

We expect you find this difficult to believe of *your man*. Some of you will think, "He's already stuck his four-inch wonder into every conceivable crevice and hole in my body, what else could he possibly want?" Some of you will scoff, "My Bill, *depraved?* Ha!" Some of you will simply close your ears to the terrifying potential of *what your man really wants*. But *all* of you will ask:

"If there's something he wants, why in the world doesn't he ask for it? The worst I can do is say *no.*"

First, it is crucial to understand that your man believes you will most certainly think his secret desires *depraved* (even if he doesn't think so himself). Why?

Consider the adage, **"Don't defecate where you eat."**

A man's mate is his spiritual sanctuary, his halo of wholesomeness, the embodiment of (so-called) ethic and (so-called) morality he would choose for himself in his finest moment. Why, for the love of God, would he deface the only pure thing in his life?

You? Pure? That's a laugh, you might think.

But it's not a laugh to him. He wouldn't be with you if he couldn't keep you up on that pedestal, safe not only from a world of disgusting men but from his own depraved desires. Yes, to your man you are an immaculate island in an ocean of excrement. And he needs you to **keep being** this island to which he can return again and again whenever he feels contaminated by the dirt of the world he was playing in when he was away from you. And because he thinks *you* want *him* to be as clean and immaculate as *he* wants *you* to be, he will never volunteer to bring his most depraved desires out into the open. *(Why risk being humiliated by **you** thinking him a degenerate when he is humiliated enough by **his own** self-judgment?)* This is a no-win position for him.

Therefore, it is up to you to know if there is something he wants without his having to tell you. This is obviously a thorny problem. How to probe his mind for debasement without puncturing his illusions of purity? The most extreme alternative is to offer him the act you suspect he may want and, if he accepts it (*trying to appear* reluctant), there is a high likelihood he is internally dancing a jig, rejoicing in the glorious sexual gift you have bestowed upon him and thinking, "How did she know I wanted that?" But beware, for he will not ever acknowledge that this is something he's always wanted—he will always "*reluctantly*" accept it as many times as you offer it.

So how do you figure out what to do? We're happy to report that the search for an answer is over. After years of penetrating (and often bruising) psychosexual research, **SMITH AND DOE** are proud to finally present the irrefutable mathematical formula *from which you can determine the degree to which your man currently harbors Depraved Sexual Desires* (DSS).

HOW TO DETERMINE THE DEGREE TO WHICH YOUR MAN CURRENTLY HARBORS DEPRAVED *SEXUAL DESIRES*

THE FORMULA

$$(SAD) + (PIW) \div (SI) = DSD$$

Note: (DSD = Degree of Sexual Depravity)

THE VARIABLES

(SAD) Sexual Acts Denied. This refers to the number and repetition of sexual acts he has requested you perform that you have declined to perform. These may be acts that you *did* perform at least once in the past but, for one reason or another, have decided not to perform again (at least for the present). Even if *you* do not consider the act *depraved* you must still count it. (The fact is that *he does*, or he would not only *ask* you to perform it but *repeatedly insist* that you do.)

To the best of your recollection, within the term of your sexual relationship, there are at least _____ different sexual acts he has requested that *you* have declined to perform: (use the number assignment in parentheses for your equation)

0 (0)

1 (1)

2 (4)

3 **(8)**
4 **(16)**
More than 4 **(20)**

(PIW) Position in the World. This factor refers to your man's position in society *as perceived by the rest of the world.* According to our research, the startling correlation here is that the higher a man's position in the world, the more depraved his sexual appetites. For example, through discreet interviews with female sex professionals, we learned that a CEO is more likely to request severe sexual punishments than a construction worker and a man of the cloth more likely to request toilet training than a traveling salesman.

Your man is most often perceived as a:
King *(i.e., politician or executive)* **(10)**
Bishop *(i.e., clergyman or "spiritual" person)* **(9)**
Knight *(i.e., athlete or soldier)* **(8)**
Pawn *(i.e., construction worker or minor bureaucrat)* **(7)**
Court Jester *(i.e., writer or salesman)* **(6)**
Queen *(i.e., interior decorator or Richard Simmons)* **(20)**

(SI) Self-Image. This is the way your man perceives his own place in the world. For instance, while the rest of the world perceives him as a leader, he may think of himself as a loner. Or a homely man may perceive himself as a studmuffin. Or a cowardly man a hero. The point is, although your man's depravity factor rests heavily on his position in the world, it rests even more on his own self-image; you must, therefore, divide the former by the latter.

The person who *best describes* your man's own self-image is:

Casanova (10)

Sir Lancelot (3)

King Arthur (2)

Pope John Paul (1)

Joe DiMaggio (4)

Rodney Dangerfield (6)

Bill Gates (5)

Pee Wee Herman (9)

Jesse Ventura (7)

Woody Allen (8)

SCORING

$$(SAD) + (PIW) \div (SI) = DSD$$

The *most* depraved score is 40
$$[20 + 20 \div 1 = 40]$$

The *least* depraved score is .6
$$[0 + 6 \div 10 = .6]$$

If he scored between .6–.9 (*i.e., a writer who thinks he's Casanova and has never asked for an odd sexual act*): **He's totally secure with his ability to make love, preoccupied with his work, and too conscience-driven to ask anyone to perform a sexually depraved act.**

If he scored between 1–1.9 (*i.e., a warrior who thinks he's Rodney Dangerfield and has asked for one unusual sexual act*): **He's got the conquering spirit which makes him goal-oriented toward a specific act but he thinks he**

gets too little respect to achieve it. He is therefore capable of but not obsessed with depravity.

If he scored between 2–3.5 (i.e., a boss who thinks he's Bill Gates but has only asked for one sexual act): **His ego is out of control, yet he goes to great lengths to hide his depravity from you.** Because of his exalted position he is reluctant to reveal *to you* his desire for the spanking he so richly deserves.

If he scored between 3.6–4.9 (i.e., he's a plumber who thinks of himself as Sir Lancelot and has asked for 2 sexual acts): **Watch this man closely during sex.** If he closes his eyes at least 50% of the time he is definitely picturing another woman's anus.

If he scored between 5–20 (i.e., he's a salesman who thinks of himself as King Arthur and has asked for 3 sexual acts): **He is a man with delusions of grandeur and therefore out of control.** You *must* appease him on a regular basis, even if you only engage in one of the depraved acts he has requested. Failure to do so will result in him wearing female underwear in the presence of another woman, leading to regular cross-dressing in public.

If he scored between 20–40 (i.e., he's perceived as Richard Simmons, thinks of himself as the pope and has asked for 4 or more sexual acts you won't perform): **Your man has probably already paid a prostitute to defecate on his chest.**

Meditation for the Day

"A man stranded on a desert island who will not have sex with a chicken is not man enough for me."

10

THE POLITICS OF **PREVENTION**

Our shocking research for **WHAT MEN DON'T WANT WOMEN TO KNOW** proved that fully 96.4% of all men either have cheated, are currently cheating, or believe they will cheat in the future. *(This is a fact of life. If you don't believe it, ask Sally Jesse Raphaël. Sally had **SMITH AND DOE** on her show and publicly doubted our findings. We were forced to have her conduct an experiment for our follow-up appearance to prove our validity. Two production assistants from the show, wholesome and attractive young ladies fitted with secret cameras and microphones, visited a randomly selected, upscale lounge in Manhattan, where they individually struck up conversations with various men. The approach each girl used was that she was in town for one night on business, had a hotel suite waiting upstairs with a Jacuzzi and bottle of champagne. All she wanted from the man was a sexual partner for an hour or two, after which they would never speak to or see each other again. The girls spoke to single men, married men (wearing wedding bands), and even men who had dates or girlfriends with them elsewhere in the lounge. Guess what—**SMITH AND DOE** were wrong. 96.4% of the men didn't take the bait—100% did!)*

Therefore, although your first response will probably be to grant our figures are true for men in general, you will then think, ***not* your *man***. Think again. Unless he is

chained in the basement, hopelessly gay, or pitifully dys-
functional, *it is your man!* The only rational response you
can have to our shocking research is, **"Forewarned is
forearmed."**

**The only women whose men will never cheat are those who take
a PROACTIVE approach to the problem.**

Being proactive clearly means thinking in terms of *prevention.*

There's nothing you can do about his *past* cheating, the
past is over. And we've been doing our best to equip you with
means for dealing with cheating in the present. *What concerns us right here is that frightening group of men
who will cheat in the future*—in other words, *prevention.*

As he comes upon his options for cheating, your man will
follow definite patterns, enabling you to zero in on his
thought process *as if you were him.* If you are aware of his
most tempting possibilities, you will be able to preempt
them before they become realities.

WHERE YOU WILL FIND THE WOMAN YOUR MAN IS MOST LIKELY TO CHEAT WITH

There are **THREE PRIMARY GROUPS** *of women who
present the most clear and present danger to you.* (Of
course there are others, like the one-night stands—as on
the Sally Jesse Show—or prostitutes he will gleefully
meet in such venues as business trips and bachelor parties. Those are merely fast-food fucks and present no long-
lasting danger to your actual relationship.) What we are
dealing with here in **PREVENTION** are the **groups clos-
est to you,** who therefore *most deeply threaten your rela-*

tionship. Therefore, we have divided our formula into three parts.

PART I:
THE SOCIAL CIRCLE

THE FORMULA

(SW + AD) × (APTH) = (SCP)
Note: (SCP = Social Cheating Potential)

THE VARIABLES

(SW) A Woman (or *Women)* You Both Socialize With. How many stories have you heard about men carrying on affairs with people who live twenty-eight miles down the road? *Never.* As necessity is the mother of invention, proximity is the mother of infidelity. Now think about how many stories you've heard about husbands cheating with their neighbors. Maybe not as many as men and their secretaries, but it still happens every day. Or social circles where somebody's husband and somebody else's wife are exploring sacred orifices while their hapless mates are working their tails off in the office, staring longingly at photos of their mates, smiling, while in reality he or she is chowing someone else's ass. This sometimes goes on for years before they get caught. A social venue where he encounters other attractive women on a more or less regular basis is very tempting for your man. He can flirt with another woman—or she can flirt with him—right under your nose without you thinking anything of it. Actually carrying on an affair is a little more dangerous, but if the attraction is strong, rest <u>un</u>assured, he will risk anything for the sex. Select from the following the statement that *most closely describes* your man:

Whenever our social group gets together, my man . . .

Sticks by my side like a faithful dog. (**1**)

Is equally friendly to male and female friends. (**2**)

Usually interacts more with the women than the men. (**3**)

Seems to get along very well with one of the women, and
later mentions that you two should "set her up" because
she's such a "great girl." (**4**)

Always seems to spend time with one particular woman. (**5**)

(**AD**) **Age Difference Between Your Man and the Other Woman/Women.** This requires no explanation. Research shows that a man who cheats on you with a woman older than himself is either getting so little from you that he is acting out of desperation or is so unattractive that an old bag is all he can reel in. Statistics prove beyond any doubt whatsoever that men overwhelmingly desire younger women with whom to engage in out-of-relationship sexual forays. To arrive at the correct choice for (**AD**), *refer back to the previous element* (**SW**) and select the age difference between your man and the woman or women involved. *(If more than one woman, select the difference between his age and their* average *age.)*

Your man is ____ years older than the woman/women you have in mind.

20 or more (**1**)

15–20 (**2**)

10–15 (**3**)

0–10 (**4**)

about the same age (**5**)

(**APTH**) **Attention Paid to Him.** *"In the eyes of your man, there can never be too many women who lust for* *and want him,"* said a very wise man *(who shall remain nameless to protect his marriage)*. Therefore, your man will do everything in his power, short of covert flirtation directly in your line of sight, to curry attention and favor from women (or one woman) in your social circle. Keeping in mind the woman/women you have been zeroing in on, select the phrase that ***best describes*** the attention that she/they pay(s) to your man.

A woman or women in your social circle treat(s) your man like . . .

He's a total gentleman. (1)

He's a lovable nebbish. (2)

He's invisible *(a common ploy for hiding her affection from you)*. (3)

He needs a big hug or he'll waste away. (4)

He's hung like a whale. (5)

SCORING

(SW + AD) × (APTH) = (SCP)

Social Cheating Potential *highest* score is 125.

$[5 + 5 \times 5 = 50]$

Social Cheating Potential *lowest* score is 2.

$[1 + 1 \times 1 = 2]$

(HOLD ONTO YOUR SCORECARDS AS WE PROCEED TO PART II)

PART II:
THE WORKPLACE

THE FORMULA

$(WW + AD) \times (APTH) = (WCP)$
Note: (WCP = Workplace Cheating Potential)

THE VARIABLES

(WW) A Woman (or *Women*) He Works With. Life at the office or on the job is a highly dangerous place for your man to be without you. As we so emphatically stated in our previous book: *"If you saw your man at the office or on the job when you are not present, you would become physically ill."* This is a place where temptation always, without fail, rears its ugly head. If your man has any attractive female underlings where he works, be warned! Keep his interaction with these women under careful surveillance in all ways possible. (For more information on these procedures, consult **"The Five Basic Points of Workplace Safety"** in **SMITH AND DOE**'s **WHAT MEN DON'T WANT WOMEN TO KNOW.**) We know that it's difficult to gauge his interaction with coworkers without being physically present, so we've made it easier by offering the following choices—select the one that ***best describes*** his most recent attitude:

When it comes to his work, my man . . .
Tells me to stop by and visit him any time. **(1)**
Displays a horrible reluctance to be apart from me. **(2)**
Doesn't like to discuss the women he works with. **(3)**
Takes more care with his grooming and dressing
than ever before. **(4)**

Occasionally comes home with female hairs, scents, or cosmetics clinging to his clothing. **(5)**

(AD) Age Difference Between Your Man and the Other Woman/Women. Use the same method to select **(AD)** as you employed in *PART I*.

> **Your man is _____ years older than the woman/women he works with:**
> 20 or more **(5)**
> 15–20 **(4)**
> 10–15 **(3)**
> 0–10 **(2)**
> about the same age **(1)**

(APTH) Attention Paid to Him. Once again, since you are not with him at work, you can't exactly judge how much attention women pay to him. You can, however, take a stab at how much he seems to **need from them.** Normally, a man who spends more time at his job is more successful. The problem evolves as the more successful he is, the more attractive he is to the women who work with him, ergo the more attention they pay him. The flip side of this is that by establishing the "alibi" of a strong work ethic, your man is capable of using that supposed "ambition" to climb the corporate ladder into someone else's skintight pants. To determine how much attention your man is receiving from women at work, select the choice that *most closely* approximates the hours he elects to spend working:

> **Lately, your man seems to attend more . . .**
> Lunch meetings. **(1)**
> Early morning meetings. **(2)**

Late-hour meetings. (3)
Cocktail meetings. (4)
Office parties. (5)

SCORING

(WW + AD) × (APTH) = (WCP)

Work Cheating Potential *highest* score is 50.
$[5 + 5 \times 5 = 50]$

Work Cheating Potential *lowest* score is 2.
$[1 + 1 \times 1 = 2]$

(HOLD ONTO YOUR PART I & II SCORECARDS AS WE PROCEED TO PART III)

PART III: EX-GIRLFRIENDS

THE FORMULA

(EG + AD) × (APTH) = (EGCP)
Note: (EGCP = Ex-Girlfriend Cheating Potential)

THE VARIABLES

(EG) His Ex-Girlfriends. BEWARE! This is the most frightening group of women you will ever encounter. A man may break social, psychological, career, or even family ties with a woman, but he will always consider her in his back pocket when it comes to clandestine sex. Beware of every woman with whom he has ever had sex or a prolonged relationship. Check his Filofax, phone book, or scraps of desk paper for women listed by first names only. Check his drawers for old photos of him with girls you don't know. Be skeptical of every "friendship" he carries on with an ex-girlfriend. If he thinks you are not paying attention to one of these women he will attempt to finagle a sexual encounter with her. *NO MAN MAINTAINS A FRIENDSHIP WITH AN ATTRACTIVE EX-GIRLFRIEND WITHOUT SECRETLY HARBORING A DESIRE TO HAVE SEXUAL RELATIONS WITH HER AGAIN.* And although this may already have happened and/or be happening, realize and understand that in this situation the man ALWAYS wants the girl. (And at the very, very least, he'll think of her while he's having sex with you, longing for the days of yesteryear when he did _____ with her).

Why are ex-girlfriends so popular with cheaters? Because it is comfortable for both of them. If he's in a relationship and she is too, they are sure enough about each other not to fear betrayal. This is critical because, as we have proven, *"The only reason a man will restrain himself from cheating is fear of getting caught."* In addition to that, because an ex-girlfriend is a *one-nighter* and requires *no commitment* from him, therefore causing him to feel *no guilt whatsoever,* she is as good and as safe as a hooker—and she saves him hundreds of dollars to boot. The friendship is like a secret handshake that implies, "At any given moment we could duck into that closet and no one would ever know, even though your mate is ten feet away." Select the comparison that *best describes* your man's ex-girlfriend status:

Ex-girlfriends are like ____ to your man:
Catnip *(finds them irresistible)* (5)
Glue *(can't set himself free from them)* (4)
Hypnotists *(mesmerized by them)* (3)
Sharks *(has to fight them off)* (2)
Pepper spray *(wants no part of them)* (1)

(AD) Age Difference Between Your Man and the Other Woman/Women. Use the same method to select **(AD)** as you employed in *PARTS I and II*.

Your man is ____ years older than his ex-girlfriends.
20 or more (1)
15–20 (2)
10–15 (3)
0–10 (4)
about the same age (5)

(APTH) Attention Paid to Him. Your man is more likely to contact his ex-girlfriends than they are to contact him, but once that contact is made, they have no compunctions about getting their "friendship" afloat again. Here's where you get to use all the information he's innocently passed on to you regarding his past relationships.

From everything he's ever told you, his ex-girlfriends treated him like a . . .
Piece of steaming dung. (1)
Well-scuffed soccer ball. (2)
Teddy bear. (3)
VIP. (4)
Stud-Muffin. (5)

SCORING

$(EG + AD) \times (APTH) = (EGCP)$

Ex-Girlfriend Cheating Potential is *highest* at 50.
$[5 + 5 \times 5 = 50]$

Ex-Girlfriend Cheating Potential is *lowest* at 2.
$[1 + 1 \times 1 = 2]$

At this point you have three scores: (SCP), (WCP), and (EGCP). To accommodate the varying risk factors, perform the following additions:

$$(EGCP) + 15$$
$$(WCP) + 10$$
$$(SCP) + 5$$

__Whichever score comes out HIGHEST is the group from which he has cheated, is currently cheating, or will cheat in the future.__

☺

Meditation for the Day

"A man who is working out regularly is a man who wants to look good for other opportunities. A truly satisfied man is an out-of-shape man."

11

YOUR MAN'S "PROPENSITY TO PACK YOUR BEST FRIEND" *QUOTIENT*

Unfortunately for women (or fortunately, depending on your tolerance for mental anguish), most men harbor their sexual fantasies deep in the recesses of their conscious mind, never to be revealed. To make matters worse, most women think they know their mate's deepest, darkest desires. Why do they think this? *Because their man swore, promised, and gave his most solemn oath that they do and that it's the truth!*

But men would sooner cut off their genitals with a dull butter knife than tell their mate what they *really* want in bed. One of your man's most disgusting fantasies (aside from packing your mother, sister, or daughter from another marriage) is having sex with your best friend. Even a semi-attractive girlfriend brings up images in his mind he is genetically incapable of resisting. So how do you know if *your man* fantasizes about having sex with your best friend? **SMITH AND DOE**'s formula below will give you an idea of what we call his:

"PROPENSITY TO PACK THE BEST FRIEND" QUOTIENT

In layman's terms, this formula will tell you how likely or unlikely—(but getting *that* result is, well, unlikely)—your man is to harbor dangerous secret fantasies.

However, before we reveal what you're likely to see as *a horrible truth*, remember that all men have fantasies—it's just that they don't want to hurt your feelings (or cause you to throw yourself headfirst off a twenty-story building) by telling you that while they're having sex with you they're fantasizing about someone you may already be jealous of. Men realize that telling you something like this will only make matters worse and put you on RED ALERT, searching for any indicator of this "secret" desire manifesting itself in reality.

For example, if your man has confessed that he loves huge breasts, but you have small breasts, he will have condemned himself to a life of never being able to stare at women's huge breasts, because you will constantly be searching for this type of behavior (and will crush him like a bug if you catch him).

THE FORMULA

$$(H) + (EC) + (PG) + (BM) \div (WF) = (PTPBF)$$

Note: If you cannot find an appropriate response for each variable, approximate your answer according to the options given.

THE VARIABLES

The first factor in this equation is **H (Honesty Factor). H** is a function of how honest your man has been in matters *that have resulted in his own embarrassment and/or regret.* This is the only true measure of a man's honesty: If he tells the truth and it makes him look bad, then it's really the truth (or, if he's a really shady character, the embarrassing story is masking something far, far worse). *Anything else your man says should be entirely disregarded as bullshit.* In order to arrive at the number that will be plugged in for this variable, ask yourself the following question:

When your man was accused of something and confessed to it, it involved:
Leaving the toilet seat up. (1)
Forgetting to do something you told him to. (2)
Finances. (3)
His supposed itinerary while on a "business trip." (4)
Potential evidence of unfaithfulness on his part. (5)

The second variable, **EC (Embarrassing Confession)**, involves the things your man has told you—whether about his past, present, or future—that are just plain embarrassing. These types of confessions are usually good windows into the dark side of your man, because rarely does a man tell these things with the intention of manipulating his mate or gaining anything except a hearty dose of regret once the words have left his lips. The bottom line is that if your man tells you something that is embarrassing and raises issue with his manhood, sexual proclivities, and/or character, you should file it away, because it can tell you a lot. To arrive at this variable's value, answer the following question:

Did the most embarrassing thing your man ever told you involve:
Embarrassing clothing or hairstyle as an ignorant and headstrong youth. (1)

A hideous girl that he once sexually interacted with in a drunken stupor. (2)

Harboring interest in something embarrassing, i.e., Barry Manilow. (3)

Masturbation, pornography, or other sexual *faux-pas* stories. (4)

Being secretly attracted to men. (5)

PG (Past Girlfriends) is a very important part of this equation. Women underestimate the knowledge that is to be gleaned from the analysis of past girlfriends' physical attributes. You can tell what attracts your man (if all his past girlfriends have big breasts, and you have small breasts, your man is spending an inordinate amount of time longing for big breasts but tolerating yours since you bring something else to the table and aren't worth jettisoning just yet for the huge-racked intern that just started working down the hall). If your man used to only date blondes and you're a brunette, rest assured he's still more attracted to blondes.

With regard to your man's past girlfriends, which of the following applies?

They all seem to be the same type, and I fit the same description. (1)

They all treated him like garbage. (2)

They are all different types, and he likes to keep in touch with all of them. (3)

He did something sexual with all of them that I won't do with him. (4)

They are all the same type, and look nothing like me. (5)

I don't know, he's never previously had a girlfriend. (10)

BM (Bating Material) is another important factor in your man's SNA (as opposed to DNA, SNA is your man's ***Scum-oxyribonucleaic Acid,*** which is a strand of proteins that, when analyzed at **SMITH AND DOE**'s lab, provides a clear picture of your man's sexual character). The material that your man masturbates to, whether in magazine or video format, is a telltale indicator of what turns him on.

Does his bating material . . .

Fit the standard bill, nothing fetish-like
or out of the ordinary? (**1**)
Seem normal, but all involves the same
type of woman? (**2**)
Seem normal, but all involves the same type of woman who
looks nothing like you? (**3**)
Consist of very young women
(who look like teenagers)? (**4**)
Consist of very young boys? (**5**)
Revolve around a sexual act that you won't let him do to
you? (**6**)
Involve the release and/or smearing of fecal matter? (**10**)

The final factor in this equation is your man's **WF (Weirdness Factor)**. This involves just how out-there your man's secret desires actually are. Remember that if your man is telling you sexual fantasies, desires, or needs that seem strange to you, you are only hearing the most sugar-coated of thoughts. His true, deep, dark secrets would make you violently ill, projectile vomiting as you retch with the horrid realization that your man is a freak of nature. ***And the worst part of it is that he's probably totally normal by other men's standards.***

When your man has told you about sexual fantasies, stories of his past, or described things he wants to do to you,

They seem normal and are nothing that you found
weird in any way. (5)

They seem pretty normal, there are a few things
that concern you a little, but nothing you
wouldn't live with. (4)

They seem to revolve around bringing another girl
into the relationship. (3)

They seem to revolve around bringing another guy
into the relationship. (2)

You wouldn't know, he never talks to you about
that kind of stuff. (1)

SCORING

The highest achievable score is PTPBF = 30. *If your man scored anything near this, you should panic and panic now.* There is little you can do to repair the damage that has already been done, but if you are willing to go forward in your relationship knowing that your man has probably sexually interacted with your coworkers, friends, and relatives, go forward knowing the truth. Trying to stop such activities in the future will prove utterly fruitless.

If he scored 20–25, he's in the RED ZONE. *You need to be on what SMITH AND DOE describe as RED ALERT,* constantly searching for indications of impending infidelity.

If he scored 10–20, *he's relatively normal, and although he is undoubtedly attracted to your friends, coworkers, and relatives, he probably won't act on it.*

That is, unless alcohol is involved and you aren't present, in which case you should keep a careful eye out for pregnant friends.

If he scored under 10, *he's either a great actor, or you're either very stupid or very lucky.* This guy may actually be on the level.

If he scored less than 1, *get married immediately and stage a weekly auction of his DNA for cloning purposes.*

Meditation for the Day

"A man who laughs at my accusations is a man who takes me too lightly."

12

FORMULA TO SHOW HOW YOUR MAN'S SEXUAL PREFERENCES IMPACT HIS FINANCIAL FUTURE

When a man frees a captive genie from a bottle lying on the beach, what's the first thing he asks for: a wonderful night of sex with the woman of his dreams, or a billion dollars?

If you ask *any* man what's more important to him, sex or money, he'll think about it for a moment. Sex is important, he'll think, but without money, I won't get any sex—*so money it is!*

Every semi-conscious man learns at a very early age that the reason bald fat guys have beautiful supermodels on their arm is that their bulging wallets are as fat as their bulging guts. This knowledge in turn fuels a man's ambition, the ambition to get rich and powerful so that he, too, can have that supermodel regardless of his looks, or lack thereof.

If you're a woman, you've found yourself pleasantly on the opposite side of this equation. "Well that *sounds funny, but the reality is I don't care about money, I just want a wonderful man who loves me.*" Really? Line up 100 women with that attitude and ask them this question: "Here are two guys. They are similar in almost every way except one's insolvent and one is a billionaire. Which do you want to marry?" *Not one woman will choose the guy with no money—**not one!*** Would you?

This horrid reality is as bad for men as it is for women. It reminds us that without a strong income we're going to need a strong right hand for masturbation. The fact that a man without money has dramatically lower odds of getting a woman who isn't a beast is a painful reality with which every man is forced to live.

So let's cut to the chase: **How do you avoid the men who will never have enough money to make them worth your while?** Well, **SMITH AND DOE** have learned that by analyzing a man's sexual preferences, you can grasp a clear insight into his financial future. What the following formula will tell you is ***how likely your man is to be successful based on his sexual preferences.*** So at least you can rest at ease knowing that if your man passes with flying colors but is working at the local IHOP, maybe he'll be promoted in the near future to assistant manager.

THE FORMULA

$$FF = TS + TY + F + A + SP \div C$$

THE VARIABLES

TS (Timing of Sex): A man who wants sex in the morning is a man who isn't concentrating on the workday ahead of him. We have found that most men who are sexually active in the morning couldn't give a rat's ass about the meeting later today (which could have a bearing on whether or not you're going to trade in your '82 Chevy for something a little more recent). *So on a scale of 1–5, 1 being sexually active and 5 being a man who rarely touches you in the morning, plug in the number.*

TY (Type of Sex): A man who relishes oral sex (is there a kind who doesn't?), we mean *really* relishes oral sex, is a man who is used to being in control and having his ass kissed, watching relaxedly as others do his bidding. Same goes for a man who likes to have sex doggy style: This guy is used to closing deals and really driving the point home. A guy who likes anal sex (**with *women*, that is**) is a man who is so successful that everything's old hat; he needs something new and different. So if your man's favorite sex act is blowjobs, *put a 1 here.* Doggy style sex, a *2.* Anal sex, a *5.* And if he likes something totally bizarre or something not on this list, just leave this as *zero.*

F (Frequency of Sex): A successful man enjoys sex thoroughly, but he's got more important things to do than worry about chasing you around every time he finds himself capable of getting it up again. He is so confident and in control that he *knows* he can gain sexual release any time he wants to, so he's not in any rush. *On a scale of 1–5, 1* being a man who has sex with you every time a little blood flows into his nether regions and *5* being a guy who doesn't have sex with you every second he can, but when he does he really delivers, plug in a number.

A (Level of Adventure): An imminently wealthy man feels an inexplicable urge to try new things. Not unlike Albert Einstein doodling in beginner's math classes, a man destined for financial greatness finds mainstream things relatively boring. You may find this type of man spending an inordinate amount of time on the Internet, exploring the wealth of knowledge (not to mention porn) there. You may find this type of man reading voraciously or discussing complex ideas like most people would talk about the weather. So when your man asks for a threesome with your best friend, or some type of exotic sex, don't get mad at him; instead, **rejoice in the imminent cash that you now know is en route to your bank account!** *On a scale of 1–5, 1* being your standard missionary guy and *5* being a guy who needs to use plastic sheets 'cause things get so ugly, plug in the number.

SP (Satisfaction Principle): A wealthy-man-to-be is never satisfied. If he makes a load of money one day, within a few days he feels relatively poor and feels an urgent need to move on to the next score. He gets equally bored in bed; the same old thing just doesn't do it anymore. So if you find yourself having to spend more time and effort to sexually satisfy your man than you did a few months ago, put a *5* here. If his threshold has been relatively static, and he seems to be just as satisfied as he was a few months ago, put a *zero* here.

C (Propensity to Cuddle): A man who likes to cuddle with you resting your head on his chest is a man who is going to make millions. Because he loves you, you ask? Because he's sensitive and kind? Hell, no! It's because while you're lying there rambling on, spewing some inane banter about the trials and tribulations of your most recent hair appointment, he's thinking about the stock market. *So if your man likes to cuddle, put a 1 here. If he doesn't, put a 5 here.*

SCORING

If your man scored over 15, you are never going to have to worry about money. No matter what he's doing, the money will somehow find its way into his life and, soon thereafter, your life. Assuming you don't get the boot because he decides he wants someone younger and cellulite-free, you can look forward to a life of relaxation and riches.

If your man scored between 5–15, there's good news and there's bad news. The bad news is you can forget the yacht. The good news is you can also forget the trailer park, since this man is going to make a good living for most of his life. With the exception of those trying times when he's being sued for child support by a teenage babysitter who "claims" he had sex with her multiple times while you foolishly stood by his side in court, you will live a full and happy life, never wanting anything—except those things that cost over five figures.

If your man scored below 5, it doesn't matter what he says, what he hopes, or what he dreams. This loser is going nowhere fast, and you can rest assured that if he were a stock we'd all be selling him short. This guy was probably hung by his underwear from clothes hooks after sports when he was little, a prescient act that accurately foretold the financial horror that will become this man's life. Run and run *now,* for the longer you stay with him, the worse you will feel about leaving him when he finds out the eraser factory is closing and he's going to lose his job.

Meditation for the Day

"(YOUR MAN'S NAME)
genuinely believes he was born
to rule, and until
I can physically kick the
shit out of him, that's the way
it will stay."

13

FORMULA TO DETERMINE YOUR MAN'S SEXUAL SAFETY FACTOR AT ANY GIVEN MOMENT

In our first groundbreaking study, we determined that man exists in one of two basic states: *loaded or unloaded*; and that he spends the bulk of his waking day trying, in one fashion or another, to reach the *unloaded* state. Once he is *unloaded*, he remains in that state for a period of time which is primarily determined by his age (a man of 20 takes approximately 24 hours to become loaded again, whereas a man of 50 can take up to 72 hours). During the time he is *unloaded*, he will not be interested in sex, therefore rendering him **SAFE** from the possibility of trying to become *unloaded* with another woman. **SMITH AND DOE urge all women to NEVER SEND YOUR MAN INTO A TARGET-RICH ENVIRONMENT (i.e., the office, a neighborhood swim party) IN THE *LOADED* STATE.**

To determine *your man's* **Safety Factor (SF) at any given moment**, work out the following equation:

THE FORMULA

$$(LU) \times (F) \times (OFF \times 10) \div (ATM) = (SF)$$

THE VARIABLES

(LU) The first factor to be determined is the amount of time that has passed between your man's *last (known) unloading* **(LU) and this moment**. This is a critical number, the selection of which should be undertaken only if you are at least *80% sure* his last unloading was *with you* (or he has confessed to unloading elsewhere, i.e., via masturbation). To determine his **LU**, select the number that applies to your man.

His last unloading was . . .
1–12 hours ago **(1)**
13–24 hours ago **(2)**
25–36 hours ago **(3)**
37–72 hours ago **(4)**
more than 72 hours ago **(5)**

(F) Unloading is not as cut-and-dried a process as one might imagine. Each unloading has its own level of satisfaction. The next factor you must quantify is the *fullness* of his last unloading **(F)**. To determine **(F)**, *add the numbers* that describe his last unloading.

During or after the time of his last unloading . . .
His body went totally limp. **(1)**
He bucked like a Brahma bull. **(2)**
He moaned like a rhino in heat. **(3)**
He screamed like he was being electrocuted. **(4)**

He ejaculated two or more tablespoonsful while spasming, teetering on the brink of cardiac arrest. **(5)**

(ATM) An absolutely essential element of this equation is where he physically is *at the moment* **(ATM)** of calculating his degree of safety. Again, add each number that describes where he physically is right now.

At this very moment, he is . . .
Somewhere where there are unattached women. **(1)**
Somewhere where there is alcohol being served. **(2)**
At work. **(3)**
On a business trip. **(4)**
Somewhere other than the above, but not with you. **(5)**

(OFF) Finally, you must judge his present against his past to come up with his *overall fidelity factory* **(OFF)**. Believing fully in your own *instincts,* honestly assess the number of times you think he has actually been unfaithful to you.

He has cheated on you . . .
Five or more times **(1)**
Three times **(2)**
Two times **(3)**
Once **(4)**
Never **(5)**

*Note: The reason this number is multiplied by 10 is that the actual reality is always **ten times worse** than you think it is.*

SCORING

$$(LU) \times (F) \times (OFF \times 10) \div (ATM) = (SF)$$

The *most dangerous* score is (SF) = 75
$$[5 \times 15 \times 10 \div 10 = 75]$$

The *least dangerous* score is (SF) = 125
$$[1 \times 5 \times 50 \div 2 = 125]$$

If he scored 70–75, he could well be having sex with another woman at this very moment.

If he scored 76–85, he's most likely flirting with another woman, hoping and longing for some form of sex.

If he scored 86–110, he probably just struck out, but his intentions were thoroughly repugnant.

If he scored 111–124, the only one he's having sex with (besides you) is himself.

If he scored 124–500, you have absolutely nothing to worry about (except that he may not be a real man).

Meditation for the Day

"The primary reason (YOUR MAN'S NAME) *occasionally restrains himself from cheating can be summed up in one word: FEAR."*

14

FORMULA TO DETERMINE THE ODDS THAT YOU ARE THE BEST SEX YOUR MAN EVER HAD

Have you ever privately wondered or actually asked your man, "Am I the best sex you ever had?" *If you don't care about the answer, read no further—there's nothing we can do to prolong a doomed relationship.* But if you really *want* to be the best sex partner he's ever had, you need to analyze the entire realm of his sexuality in regard to you. If your man has already declared that you are the best sex he ever had, chances are you wondered, *Is he telling me the truth?* Or *Is he just saying that because I want to hear it?* Believe this—your man will say **anything he thinks you want to hear** to keep you where *he* wants to remain—in a constant, non-demanding, one-sided state of being perpetually unloaded.

But **really,** you ask—is it possible that a man who has bedded God knows how many women (*he'll never admit to every last hosebag and hooker*) can truly say, without reservation, that I am better than every single woman he has ever had sex with? Can I really believe I give the *best head* of all his ex-lovers? Or *scream* the most? Or *come* the most?

If you truly desire to know how you rank in his sexual pantheon, work out the formula below.

THE FORMULA

(A) + (B) + (C) = ODDS

(A) = EE + CC
(B) = GS + OC
(C) = OBF + SI

Note: We give only odds on how you rate because there is always the possibility that there is a legendary one-nighter lodged in your man's memory, a holy shrine where he worships, that nothing you do will ever replace.

THE VARIABLES

(EE) Exclamation of Ecstasy. There are many ways by which to judge how much you are turning your man on. The *Exclamation of Ecstasy* measures how close your man comes to a spiritual experience when making love to you. The combination of religious fervor and physical ecstasy is the highest point a human can reach in the achievement of total sexual satisfaction. Take, for instance, Tantric Yoga, where the essence of penetration is held until one of the participants can't stand it one more second and screams, *"Oh, sweet mother of God, fuck me sweet Jesus, I'm coming, I'm coming, I'm coming, nam yo ho renge Kyo!"* This is an excellent Exclamation of Ecstasy, although many men over 55 are lost to heart attacks in the overwhelming ecstasy of it. The simplest and most universal Exclamation of Ecstasy is, *"Oh, God! Oh, God! Oh, my God!"* If a man repeatedly exclaims these words *while having sex with you* (as opposed to while praying in church or making the best putt of his life), he has lost all sense of judgment and would choose this actual moment with you *over any one of his fondest fantasies.* In other words, by intense and repeated Exclamations of Ecstasy he unwittingly mesmerizes himself to believe that this is the single best climax he has ever had. To determine your man's **(EE),** select as many choices from below that apply to the two of you, then add them to get your number.

My man exclaims, *"Oh, God!"* . . .

Repeatedly during kissing and non-sexual touching. **(10)**
Repeatedly during sexual foreplay. **(9)**
Repeatedly during lovemaking. **(5)**
Repeatedly while preparing for his impending climax. **(3)**
Repeatedly during his actual climax. **(1)**

Note: If he is a <u>confirmed atheist</u> and still exclaims,
"Oh, God!" multiply each score by 2.

(CC) Calling of Climax. The *Calling of Climax* is man's oldest method of giving voice to sexual satisfaction. Being a totally nonverbal expression of primal pleasure, it predates verbal communication. It even predates the topic we just covered, the Exclamation of Ecstasy (which was not invented until *after* the discovery of God). When a man "calls climax," he is informing not only his partner but the entire world that he is having an orgasm. At this instant he truly believes the world is revolving around him. He thinks he is the happiest, luckiest, most blessed man on God's green earth. It is the Calling of Climax, and only the Calling of Climax, by which man establishes his highest degree of dominance over all other genders. To determine your man's (**CC**), select from the following any description that applies to him—if more than one, add them together to arrive at your number.

When my man "calls climax" he . . .
Roars like a lion. (**10**)

Screams like a hyen. (**5**)

Crows like a rooster. (**4**)

Groans like an ox. (**3**)

Shuts up like a clam. (**0**)

(**GS**) **Genital Stamina.** *(Note: This is not an aerospace company, high-ranking Greek army officer, or component of a vulva-shaped flower.)* ***Genital Stamina*** is that force which possesses your man from the onset of sexual excitation to the last thrust of climactic milking. A man who exhibits outbursts of Genital Stamina in irregular, periodic cycles is a man with Attention Deficit Disorder *when it comes to you.* When a man places a priceless value on the sexual attraction he feels for a woman, he will experience furious bursts of Genital Stamina on a repeated basis (often with the result of annoying you greatly). Even the strongest of men, when confronted by a woman who brings his stamina to ***Attention!*** like a Nazi general, is laid low by uncontrollable and repeated outbursts of Genital Stamina. The condition of Genital Stamina was first brought to public awareness by Samson, in the Bible, when he was confronted by an irresistibly voluptuous, heretically desirable, deliciously delectable work of femininity named Delilah. He literally flipped his lid. (Actually, *she* flipped his lid and gave it to the Philistines.) The point is, if you happen to be like Delilah, be prepared to deal with repeated Samson-sized bursts of Genital Stamina in return for whatever it is you want (particularly if it goes beyond the hair on his head to, say, a Ferrari). To determine the condition of your man's Genital Stamina, select the choice or choices below that apply, add the numbers if necessary, and you will have the number required to solve your equation.

My man's Genital Stamina . . .
Could recreate the moon and the stars. **(10)**
Would make a horse envious. **(9)**
Is probably of great concern to my mother. **(8)**
Probably *concerns* my mother. **(7)**
Wouldn't sustain the sex drive of a ninety-year-old basset hound. **(6)**

(OC) Orgasmic Capacity. *Orgasmic Capacity* is quite simple to measure. We are not speaking here of Orgasmic *Volume*, with which we deal in another equation. Your man's Orgasmic Capacity is the number of actual climaxes he achieves during a single, *continuous* sexual encounter, in which the two of you go at it full-bore for no less than five nor more than three thousand minutes. (Be advised that some men will fake orgasms to make you think you are sexier than you really are. And those are the *nice* guys.) Select the number you recall as being the *most* actual orgasms your man achieved during one continuous sexual encounter with you.

The most times my man has ever climaxed during a single continual sexual encounter with me is . . .
1 **(1)**
2 **(2)**
3 **(3)**

4 **(4)**
5 **(5)**
6 **(6)**
7 **(7)**
8 **(8)**
9 **(9)**
10 or more **(10)**

(OBF) Overall Bodily Fascination. This is the least exact of our judgements, since it is the most *subjective* for you to make. We understand that women (and men, too, for that matter) can appear to be rationally functioning individuals even while in the deepest and most depressive denial about the degree of loathing they have for one or more of their own body parts. Therefore, do not consider this in any way a judgment on your part. This refers specifically to **his *Overall Bodily Fascination*** with you. In order to determine the number, you must now rate him on how much attention he pays to various parts of your body. The more of your body parts that seem to engage his lust, the more his Overall Bodily Fascination is in your favor. From the twenty-five major sensual areas, select those that *you* think your man just can't get enough of. **Give each a value of one (1), then add them up and you'll have the number for your equation.**

Whenever we make love, my man is definitely fascinated with my . . .
Eyes
Ears
Nose
Mouth
Tongue
Neck
Breasts

Nipples

Arms

Hands

Navel

Pubic hair

Labia (pubic lips)

Little man in the boat (clitoris)

Vagina

Taint (the wee space down there that

'tain't your vagina and 'tain't your anus)

Outside butt cheeks

Inside butt cheeks

Anus

Sphincter

Anal canal

Thighs

Calves

Feet

Toes

(SI) Sexual Inspiration. Now we are down to the nitty-gritty. We've all heard the myth, invented by men, that size makes no difference. The reason this myth was invented was because, just as some men are short and some men are tall, some men have small penises and some men have large penises. Unfortunately, men with small penises are more egotistical and warlike, and therefore feel it necessary to manufacture myths in order to negate any failing, however small and insignificant, they might have. This is not to imply that short men have small penises and tall men have large penises. The myth that *size does not matter* has been sustained throughout time by the fact that the great majority of men do not have *large enough* penises. When they say, "Size does not matter," they are implying that something else makes up for the lack of size. This is the genesis of the ludicrous phrase, *"It's not how big it is, it's what you do with it that counts."* The concept of *"it's what you do with it that counts"* tells women that a man who is truly inspired in his sexual performance more than makes up for a laughable penis. A man's **Sexual Inspiration** is that degree of imagination, that commitment to exploration, that desire to discharge from the deepest bowels of his libido the most creative sexual acts he has ever conceived *that you inspire in him*. If you are willing to believe this compensates for anything less than nine inches (which you must believe in order to complete the equation), select from the following the **one** description that **best fits** your man's level of Sexual Inspiration.

When it comes to scaling the heights of sexual inspiration, my man could be the hero with me as the heroine in the book:

"Die Hard" (**10**)

"Naked Lunch" (**9**)

"Leave It to Beaver" (**8**)

"Lost in the Outback" (**7**)

"Willy Wonka and the Chocolate Factory" (**6**)

"A Tale of Two Titties" (**5**)

"Murder in the Rue Morgue" (**4**)

"Women Who Love Men Who Love Men" (**0**)

SCORING

$$(A) + (B) + (C) = ODDS$$

(A) = EE + CC

(B) = GS + OC

(C) = OBF + SI

If your total is 100 points, the odds are 100–1 *in your favor* that you are the best sex your man ever had.

If your total is 51 points, the odds are 51–1 in your favor.

If your total is 50 points, the chances are *EVEN* that you are the best sex your man ever had. **This is the dividing line.** *From 50 on down,* the odds are *AGAINST* you being *the best sex he ever had.*

If your total is 49 points, the odds are 49–1 *against you being the best sex he ever had.*

If you scored 25 points, the odds are 25–1 against your being the best sex your man ever had.

If your total is 1 point, the game is over, the odds are 100–1 against you.

Good luck.

Meditation for the Day

"Remember to be sure that I am the __only__ woman (YOUR MAN'S NAME) *wants to have sex with __and__ be best friends with."*

15

YOUR ACTUAL SEXUAL CA$H VALUE

PART I

FORMULA TO DETERMINE HOW MUCH YOUR MAN WOULD PAY YOU FOR SEX IF YOU WERE A PROSTITUTE (AND HE DID NOT KNOW YOU)

This is one of the most (if not *the* most) revolutionary of all the formulas you will find in this book. This equation, for the first time ever, isolates and places a definitive ***cash value*** on ***your sexual worth*** to your man by determining how much he would pay if you were a prostitute.

Why is it important for you to know this? The answer is plain as the nose on your face—if he won't pay you as much as he'd pay a prostitute something is very fishy, perhaps *too* fishy—either change your douche or ditch him for someone with deeper pockets.

In order to answer this question we have to assume your man is in love with you. If he isn't in love with you, what are you doing with him? Waiting for him to *fall* in love with you? ***Get real.***

Of course there is the possibility that he is only *in lust* with you, in which case you should make certain to get cash on the barrelhead for your services, because sooner or later he'll tire of you and invest in a newer cash cow.

Now let us assume for the sake of argument that your man is both *in love* and *in lust* with you. How is it possible to separate his love and his lust and give each a definitive value? It is not. There is no value anyone can place on love. It has been said that true love is the willingness to give up one's life for the person one loves—so can a value be placed on human life?

Though you can't separate love from lust, you can separate lust from love. And this is a story of lust.

Yes, **Lust** is quite possible to quantify. Individuals known as *prostitutes* have shown over thousands of years that lust absolutely can be quantified in terms of money. This is just one of the woefully underappreciated services prostitutes provide to society. Think of it this way: In terms of money, the world operates on *The Gold Standard*. In terms of sex, the world operates on *The Ho Standard.*

To determine *your **Ho Standard,*** work out the simple equation below.

THE FORMULA

(A) + or − (B% of A) = (C)

Note: (C) = How Much Your Man Would Pay You for Sex if You Were a Prostitute

THE VARIABLES

(A) Your Personal Sexual Value. This factor is arrived at directly from *your own sexual valuation*. As we stated earlier, in order to find a realistic figure for sex it is necessary to separate *love* from *lust*. The figure at which you arrive must be relative to sex and sex only. To accomplish this, do the following: Imagine yourself in the bar or lounge of your choice. (Depending on your current social standing the place you choose will obviously predetermine both the floor and the ceiling of your value.) Picture the single men in the place. *Rule out anyone more attractive than your man*. From the men that are left, imagine yourself striking up a conversation in which you determine that he finds you attractive enough (or is horny enough) to pay you right there and then for sex. You are going to spend one hour with him during which you will perform only rubberized oral and vaginal sex. He asks you how much it will cost. **YOUR KEY CONSIDERATION AT THIS POINT IS THAT *YOU ARE BROKE AND CAN SERIOUSLY USE THE MONEY.***

You tell him the hour of sex will cost him . . .

Less than $100

$100

$200

$300

$400

$500

$1,000

Any figure over $1,000

(B) A Prostitute's Sexual Value to Your Man. Imagine your man alone in the same social level of bar or lounge as you just pictured yourself, but in another city. Say he's on a business trip. A woman, *no less attractive than you (meaning she can be much more attractive than you, but no less attractive than you),* approaches him. He discovers she is for sale and asks her how much it will cost. (As in the previous case, he will get one hour of rubberized oral and vaginal sex for his money.) She has a figure in her head that she wants to get—it is *the same figure you determined that you would ask for.* But when he asks how much it will cost, she answers by asking him to make an offer. Knowing your man, how much would he offer to pay her, *assuming he is determined not to let her get away?*

If he does not know the figure she has in mind, would he offer . . .
Thirty percent more than her asking price?
Twenty percent more than her asking price?
Ten percent more than her asking price?
Her asking price?
Thirty percent less than her asking price?
Twenty percent less than her asking price?
Ten percent less than her asking price?

SCORING

$$(A) + or - (B\% \text{ of } A) = (C)$$

METHODOLOGY

Take the number you came to for (A), then add or subtract the appropriate percentage in (B), and you will know.

PART II

*HOW MUCH YOUR MAN WOULD PAY YOU TO PER-
FORM THE SPECIFIC SEXUAL ACT WHICH YOU
FIND MOST REPULSIVE IF YOU WERE A PROSTI-
TUTE (AND HE DID NOT KNOW YOU)*

Together with the preceding equation, this formula completes your knowledge of your actual worth to your man for one hour of sex. The difference between the two is that this *pushes* the envelope while the former just *opened* it. Here you discover the ***absolute highest value*** you place on your sexual worth to him, and the ***absolute highest dollar*** he places on the same thing. With this knowledge you will know exactly how far sex will take you in your relationship with your man.

THE FORMULA

(A) + or – (B% of A) = (C2)

Note: (C2) = How Much Your Man Would Pay You to Perform the Specific Sexual Act Which You Find Most Repulsive if You Were a Prostitute (and He Did Not Know You)

THE VARIABLES

(A) Your Personal Sexual Value. Here again we are looking for your personal view of your sexual value, taken one step further. After you and the man in the bar have agreed on a price, he then asks you to perform the sexual act which is most repulsive to you—something you have done at least once in your life—anal sex, swallowing semen, golden showers, whatever. Each of us has some sexual act we find most repulsive. Whatever yours is, that's what the man in the bar asks you to do. Since you have already committed to going with him (and you are broke, and all the other available men have left the bar), you must give him a price you think he can live with but isn't insulting to you.

On top of our already agreed upon price, the repulsive sexual act will cost him . . .

Less than $100

$100

$200

$300

$400

$500

$1,000

Any figure over $1,000

(B) A Prostitute's Sexual Value to Your Man. Once again imagine your man alone in the bar and a woman *no less attractive than you* approaches him. This time they settle on a price but he is not finished. He asks her to perform that extra sexual act, the one which you find repulsive. She tells him to make an offer. Knowing your man, how much would he offer to pay her, ***assuming he is determined to get her to do that repulsive thing (basically because you will not do it for him).***

Not knowing the figure she has in mind to do the nasty thing, would he offer . . .

Thirty percent more than her asking price?

Twenty percent more than her asking price?

Ten percent more than her asking price?

Her asking price?

Thirty percent less than her asking price?

Twenty percent less than her asking price?

Ten percent less than her asking price?

SCORING

(A) + or − (B% of A) = (C2)

METHODOLOGY

Take the number you came to for (A), then add or subtract the appropriate percentage in (B), and you will know *the amount of cash money your man would pay you to perform the specific sexual act which you find most repulsive if you were a prostitute (and he didn't know you).*

Meditation for the Day

"A man leaving on a business trip who doesn't seem to know his itinerary is a man who doesn't want his itinerary known."

16

HOW TO DETERMINE WHETHER OR NOT YOUR MAN SECRETLY WANTS YOU TO INSERT YOUR FINGERS OR INANIMATE OBJECTS INTO HIS RECTUM

Before we begin, realize that almost no man will admit that the results of this test are correct. However, throw a finger or two in his ass and you'll probably get little resistance. Why? Because most men, as much as it pains them to admit it, enjoy a certain amount of attention paid to their sphincters. In order to understand this phenomenon more clearly, think of this: ***What is the difference between a gay man and a straight man? Simply the mental preference of what turns them on; straight men are turned on by women, and gay men by other men. There is no physical difference between the two.*** Gay men are not born with some special anal nerve endings that make anal sex more pleasurable for them than for straight men. So the fact that a gay man can derive so much pleasure from this rectal revelry tells you that your man is also capable of enjoying such pleasures; it's simply a matter of how far and with how many fingers.

THE FORMULA

$$NAP = T + CY + F + CH + AI + M + HQ \times FA$$

Note: Your man's secret need for anal penetration = Taint + Chowing You + Finger + Chowing Him + Anal Insert + Music + Homophobe Quotient × Finger in the Ass

THE VARIABLES

Taint: The "taint," the space between your man's penis and ass ('tain't the ass and 'tain't the penis), is an important erogenous zone that can help you determine whether or not your man wants you going farther and further. Test this area by using your tongue during your next bout of oral sex. If your man seems to enjoy this, put a *1* here. If he panics and asks you, "What in God's name are you doing!?" put a *zero* here.

Chowing You: If your man has shown an interest in licking your sphincter, there is a high likelihood he wants and/or would enjoy the same. **SMITH AND DOE** have determined (well, actually Doe did most of *this* research) that men are either "anal" or not; there's no real in-between. You will rarely find a guy who will chow every asshole he can find, but if a girl tries to do it to him he'll scream, "What kind of man do you think I am!?" So if your man has chowed the brown eye, put a *1* here. If he's never ventured beyond the box, a *zero*.

Finger: If you have ever braved the anus far enough to try putting a fingertip or finger in and you've been met with little or no resistance, your man is practically screaming at you, "FOR THE LOVE OF GOD DO THAT ALL THE TIME, AND HARDER!" Men are shy about discussing this, and aren't likely to say, "Hey, you know what? I'm no fag but how about taking your vibrator and trying to shove it up there too?" It just doesn't happen. So if your finger's been accepted there like a long lost family member, a *1* goes here. If not, *zero*.

Chowing Him: This is an act reserved for only the most sexual of women. A woman brave enough to chow a man's hairy ass is worthy of the Congressional Medal of Ass-Chowing Honor. In most cases this is more dangerous than storming Normandy Beach, since men are far less caring about their genital cleanliness than women. As a matter of fact, men have been known to happily let a woman chow, knowing that they just sat on the toilet for an hour after returning from an all-you-can-eat corn and nuts meal (and he only wiped a couple of times). So if you've chowed him and he liked it, a *1* goes here. If you chowed him and he didn't, *zero*.

Anal Interest: As we said, men are usually either "anal" or not, so if you find your man constantly badgering you for anal sex, there is a strong likelihood he'd be interested in some anal play (of a more gentle nature—see bonus formula on page 112). So if your man's constantly trying to plunge your cable-layer, put a *1* here. If he's never wanted to pummel the brown eye, a *zero*.

Music: If your man listens to Barry Manilow, Abba, or Kenny G, put a *five* here.

Homophobe Quotient: This mathematical variable can have the unfortunate effect of rendering this entire exercise moot. A man's homophobe quotient is the level to which he fears and/or hates gays. His level of homophobia, while a personal issue he has a right to believe in, nonetheless has a strong bearing on whether or not you'll be able to get anything in his ass under any circumstances. You see, if your man is extremely homophobic, but at the same time secretly would love a large, prickly cucumber up his ass, he will NEVER, EVER admit this or allow this to happen because he would see himself as becoming that which he professes to hate. So, on a scale of *1–10*, *1* being the most homophobic and *10* being the least, plug the number in.

Finger in the Ass: If your man has put his finger in your butt more than once, put a *1* here. Otherwise it's a *zero*.

THE ANSWERS TO THIS PROBING QUESTION

If your man scored 15–20, he's open, ready, willing, and winking. You could put a small Volkswagen bug in this guy's ass and not only would he accept it, he'd push back. You can even throw the lubricant out for this guy, he needs the friction just to get some sensation.

If your man scored 10–15, he's probably going to like it. Be gentle; he's a newcomer, but once it grows on him he'll want it growing *in* him. If the first couple tries are successful and you don't send him to the hospital, there's a high likelihood this guy is going to eventually want you to throw on a strap-on and start packin'.

If your man scored 0–10, you couldn't get this guy's ass open with pliers. It's a miracle this guy can take dumps, because his ass can only open to the radius of a pinhole. Don't even bother trying with this one, he's hopeless, but that's not the bad news. The bad news is he's probably a closet flaming fag, yearning for the biggest crane he could possibly find to pummel his sphincter like the world was going to end tomorrow.

BONUS: ANAL PENETRATION FORMULA

Now that you know your man wants something in his butt, it begs the next logical questions: how far and how much? **SMITH AND DOE**, through hundreds of hours of clinical research, have determined that there is a simple way to tell exactly what your man wants:

$$AP = WYL \div 3$$

Note: **Anal Penetration = What You Like, divided by three.**

What does this mean? Well, if your man puts a full finger in your butt, then he wants one third of a finger, at most. If your man puts a vibrator in your butt, he wants the tip of the vibrator in his butt.

This formula applies not only to the size of the objects but to the speed at which they are applied. If your man pumps your butt at the speed of light, he wants his pumped at the speed of sound. It's a simple formula, really, but it works.

Meditation for the Day

"A man who suddenly starts clothing his package in revealing Calvin Klein briefs is a man who is gift-wrapping it for somebody else."

17

FORMULA TO DETERMINE THE PERCENTAGE OF TIME YOUR MAN IS THINKING OF OTHER WOMEN WHILE HE IS MAKING LOVE TO YOU

We all take for granted that fantasies are part and parcel of sex. And we also know it's *not only men* who fantasize. Yes, women do it, too, and if men knew what women were fantasizing they would run screaming from the bedroom. Therefore, in order to keep the human race procreating, we will not deal with those horrors.

Instead, we will focus on *men's* fantasies. You might be under the impression your guy always fantasizes about beautiful models and *Baywatch* babes. **Nothing could be further from the truth.** First and foremost, your man fantasizes about previous sexual conquests, usually involving some forbidden part of that conquest's anatomy. Second to that, however, your man's fantasies run to those females he actually feels he can score with when he's at his best and Lady Luck is with him: the counter girl at McDonald's, your downstairs neighbor, his supervisor's secretary, the bank teller with a nervous tic (who he believes is winking at him). These are the women who flood his mind while he's flooding you.

But **WHO he fantasizes about while making love to you** is not as important as **HOW MUCH OF THE TIME he's fantasizing.** If he's *"with"* some other woman more than 50% of the time spent in direct sexual contact with you, you're in trouble. The problem boils down to this: **If he's absent more than half the time, his mental drift will most certainly become a physical drift.**

There are exceptions to this rule. It does not apply to a man who fantasizes the **unsexiest** thing he can think of in order to prolong his erection and stave off premature ejaculation. This type of fantasizing is an old trick passed on from fathers to sons. The most popular male fantasy of the '50s was Willie Mays, who unwittingly prevented more premature ejaculations than extra base hits. (Although fantasies of ugly men **and** sexy women are designed to prevent loss of erection, unless he spends more time with Willie Mays than the McDonald's counter girl, at least he's not a *mo.*) The important figure here is **the percentage of time he spends without you. If you are not the person he's fucking in his mind at least 50% of the time, you won't be the person he's fucking in his bed 100% of the time.** It is therefore incumbent upon you to work out the following equation to determine if you're in the **fantasy danger zone.** If you are, immediately *let him know* that *you know*, before the fantasy gets all too real.

THE FORMULA

100% (TML) – (EC) – (SP) = (% TTML)

Note: 100% (TML) = 100% of Time Making Love to You; (% TTML) = Percent of Time Thinking of Other Women While He Is Making Love to You

THE VARIABLES

(EC) Percent of the time his eyes are closed while making love to you. Obtaining this number will take all your concentration. It requires you to keep your eyes on him from first arousal through final climax. If he is a fat, hairy pig and you married him for his money it's no big deal—close your eyes and think about **SMITH AND DOE**. But if he is your one true love and drives you sexually wild, you will have to resist those moments of pure ecstasy where nothing exists but your climax so that you can watch him to accurately gauge the percentage of time his eyes have been closed. Subtract the percentage that applies to your man from **(TML)**.

During sex, my man's eyes are closed approximately . . .

10% of the time

20% of the time

30% of the time

40% of the time

50% of the time

(SP) His Sexual Past. The more diverse your man's sexual past, the greater his library of memories to relive while he is having sex with you. This doesn't refer to pure numbers. It's the *variety* of sex partners that counts. If all his partners were Playboy Bunnies he's not as dangerous as someone who had fewer partners but spanned the gap between Playboy Bunnies and Hollywood Boulevard transvestite hookers. The latter supplies him with an unending parade of bizarre experiences to relive in sexual fantasies while making love to you. Add the numbers that apply to your man and subtract the total from **(TML)**.

My man's sexual past includes . . .
Virgins **(10)**
Underage girls **(9)**
Girls of different races **(5)**
Girls with 38-D racks and beyond **(4)**
Spinners (*girls under 5 feet tall and less than 100 pounds*)
(3)
Girls without gag reflexes **(2)**
Girls with ravenous sphincters **(11)**

SCORING

$$100\% \text{ (TML)} - \text{(EC)} - \text{(SP)} = (\% \text{ TTML})$$

(TTML) Total time making love to you without thinking of other women is *highest* at 90%

$$[100\% - 10\% - 0\% = 90\%]$$
This means he is thinking of you 90% of the time.

(TTML) Total time making love to you without thinking of other women is *lowest* at 6%

$$[100\% - 50\% - 44\% = 6\%]$$
This means he is thinking of other women 94% of the time.

Meditation for the Day

"If (YOUR MAN'S NAME) *is masturbating more than twice a week, I'd better find out what I am not giving him sexually that he really wants."*

18

FORMULA FOR **DETECTING LIES** ABOUT YOUR MAN'S SEXUAL PAST

Let's cut right to the chase and begin with this maxim:

NO MAN TELLS THE ENTIRE TRUTH ABOUT HIS SEXUAL HISTORY. EVER!

What man wants you to know he had unprotected sex with a Mexican hooker who, after the alcohol wore off, he realized may have been a man?

Who wants their girlfriend to know that he's hit on every stripper he found attractive and offered "whatever it takes" to get them to go home with him?

What man in his right mind would ever admit to his girlfriend that he truly feels in his heart that he could be harboring the AIDS virus?

Once you understand that your man is in fact like every other man, and as such will never reveal his deepest secrets of his dark past, you can begin to approach this equation with the level of objectiveness it requires to determine **HP**, the Horrors of His Past.

THE FORMULA

$$HP = CC + PA + XQ + BB \div VD \times HU$$

THE VARIABLES

CC (Cleanliness Claim): This variable is defined as the way your man has characterized his sexual past. For example, if your man is fat and ugly, and claims to have been nearly celibate his whole life, you probably tend to believe him. But if your man's attractive, and claims to have a pristine past that consists of few if any one-nighters, no prostitutes, and never, ever a threesome, you know he's full of crap.

So determine this variable, on a scale of **1–10, 1** being an honest rendition of a ho-filled past and **10** being a claim of a perfect, cleanly past with no shocking sexual stories to recount.

> *Note:* **If your man is in fact disgustingly unattractive and claims to have been perfectly clean, give him a *1* for this variable.**

PA (Past Admissions): *After three books and countless hours of counseling we truly hope we've ingrained the following adage into the female psyche:* **ANYTHING YOUR MAN ADMITS TO IS 10% OF THE TRUTH.** Conversely, the truth is 900% worse than what he's told you.

So on a scale of **1–10**, if your man has admitted something minor, give him a **1.** If he's admitted something major and shocking, give him a **10,** because if that's what he's *admitting* to you, the truth would make you choke on your own vomit.

XQ (Ex Quotient): *If every girl you meet with your man seems to have some form of sexual history with him, and if you are only told about this when you actually meet the girl, then you can rest assured there is a virtual toilet bowl full of secrets that you will never know about.*

Make this variable a number from **1–10, 1** being if this type of thing never happens and **10** if it seems to happen all the time.

BB (Black Book): *Take out his address book at some point when he's not around.* Look through the names. **Every name you see that is only a first name is a one-night sexual conquest.** That's the bad news. *The worse news is that he's kept the name and number in the hopes of rekindling the flame at some point while you're out of town.*

Make this variable a number from **1–10.** If he has no first names, make this a **1.** A lot, make it a **10. BONUS:** If you find a lot of pager numbers next to the first names, make this number a **20** (one-namers with pager numbers are either strippers or prostitutes).

VD (Venereal Disease): *If your man admits to past diseases, not only does he have a propensity to have unprotected sex with dirty girls, but he has the gall to think that you won't someday read our books and learn that what he's actually admitting to you is only the tip of the iceberg.* Any man who has admitted to a venereal disease is a man who is harboring much worse. If he admits to the disease, make this **1**; no disease admission, make this a **2. BONUS:** If you catch him lying about having a disease (he said he had none but you found out otherwise), make this a **0.5.**

HU (Hang-ups): *If your man's phone rings often and it's "just a hang-up," it's actually a girl that he had sex with and didn't call back.* If your man gets a lot of these, make this a **2**. If he doesn't get any hang-ups, make this a **1**.

SCORING

If your man scored between 1–10, he has been as honest about his sexual past as a man can be. That means he's told you about 30% of the truth; consider yourself lucky.

If your man scored between 20–40, your man has only told you the truth when he's been forced to, or when he knew that if he lied it would eventually come out. You are briefed on a need-to-know basis. Nothing will ever be volunteered.

If your man scored between 40–60, he takes his chances. He will never tell you anything truthful about his sexual past unless you happen to fall upon information too powerful to deny. Only then will he 'fess, and he will do so nonchalantly, as if it meant nothing and as if he could barely remember the occurrence. In reality, he probably masturbated thinking about it the night before, while having sex with you.

If your man scored over 60, he is a disease-ridden skank-bucket that literally has spent his life having sex with every girl he possibly can. This man probably got beaten up a lot during grade school and was quite probably a victim of acne and after-school wedgies. He has spent the latter years of his life making up for those horrible days by having sex with every woman he can, regardless of whether or not he has to pay for it. You will never know the truth of this man's past, but trust us, the truth's a lot closer to Wilt Chamberlain than Pat Robertson.

Meditation for the Day

"A man who launders his own clothes is a man who wants to see with his own eyes that the evidence went down the drain."

19

HOW TO DETERMINE IF YOUR MAN HAS A HIDDEN **PORNO** COLLECTION

Few women will ever understand the importance of porn in a man's life, the need for which ranks fourth after food, water, and actual, real-live sex.

Porn is a way for your man to essentially cheat without cheating, as many times as he wants, with no risk of getting a disease or any repercussions from you in the event of discovery (other than a severe dose of embarrassment).

With porn, men can choose which women they want to do it with, which sexual acts they want to perform, and they can do it as many times as they want, as many times a day as they want, and if they didn't think something went well the first time, they can simply hit the REWIND button!

Most important, there's no need to "court" the women or cuddle with them after you've had your orgasm, **and the entire date costs about $3.00!**

Starting to get the picture?

It is also known amongst men that there is no man who does not harbor a secret stash of porn somewhere in his homestead or, if he's always with his girlfriend,

somewhere outside of the house. The depths to which men will sink to hide these stashes would shock you beyond measure. Some men brave rat-infested attics, hide tapes under floorboards, carpets, or clothing. Some go the "obvious" route, which is to hide them in plain sight, thinking you would never search for a porn movie amongst his "regular" films.

Whatever the *modus operandi,* the porn exists. Whether or not your man has elected to keep it in the house is another story. Is he a "renter" or an "owner"? You make the call regarding his **PC**, his Porn Collection, with:

THE FORMULA

$$PC = T + B + S + SA + A + I \times NT \div VS$$

THE VARIABLES

T (Trunk): If your man has a trunk in his house that is locked, that you do not have the ability to open, put a **1** in for this variable. If he doesn't, a **zero**. A trunk that can only be opened by your man is a veritable mother lode of porn.

B (Briefcase): Does your man have a briefcase he "never uses"? If so, ask him to open it. He won't because it's full of porn. Classic, "never-fails" porn that he can call upon anytime he needs a "sure thing." If he has one of these, put a **1** here. If not, another **zero**. **BONUS:** If you get this briefcase open and all the girls in the magazines and/or movies look nothing like you, put a . . . actually, forget putting a number in here. Might as well just kill yourself.

S (Safe): Does your man own a safe that he claims keeps all his "important" documents, like the deed to his home and his life insurance paperwork? Ever wonder why you've never been offered the combo or the key? He's not lying, those documents *are* in there—*if he can find them amongst the layers of porn magazines and videos, that is.* If he's got a safe, put a **1** here; if not, another **zero**.

SA (Secret Area): Is there a part of your home your man seems to keep all to himself? Is there a little storage closet so full of garbage he knows you'd never so much as open it? If a place like this exists, he's using it to store porn; put a **1** here. If there's no place like this, a **zero**.

A (Attic): Attics are prime porn storage locations. No woman will brave a dark, musty attic to look for anything, ever. The fear of rats, spiders, and other horrifying vermin is simply too overpowering to allow a venture into that room. It's just as scary for guys; the difference is they'd climb Everest if there was a good porn at the top. If he has an attic, put a **1** here; if not, a **zero**.

I (Internet): Nowadays men don't have to walk up to their friendly neighborhood video counter and hand their daughter's teenage friend four gangbang pornos for rental. Nowadays they can do it in the privacy of their own home via the Internet. If your man has no business on the Internet but spends an inordinate amount of time in his computer room, alone, typically while you're up in the bedroom, put a **1** here; if he doesn't, a **zero**. **BONUS:** If your man comes into the bedroom after spending a lot of quality time with the computer and you try to sexually arouse him but he makes up some excuse why he can't have sex, you can stop this test right now. Your man was masturbating to stuff he downloaded off the Internet.

NT (Name Test): Find out the names of a couple of the biggest porn stars. Walk up to your man and out of nowhere tell him that you met a porn star named "____" today. If his face registers total and utter confusion and he truly seems to have no idea what or who you are talking about, put a **1** here. If he smiles, or is in any way not caught off guard by this, put a **2** here.

VS (Video Store): If your man has a membership at a video store you've never been to, put a **0.5** here. How do you find this out? Ask him to rent a movie on his way home. Check the movie box. If it's rented from a place you've never been to, put a **0.5** here. If it's rented from your local neighborhood shop that he takes you to, he's still not off the hook. Check his wallet for membership cards. If he's clean, give him a **1**, but check thoroughly. Why use a different store? No man wants to walk into the video store where he usually checks out porn vids and have the clerk either recognize him by name in front of his mate or, in the worst-case scenario, rent a normal video, hear a computer beep, and have the clerk say, "Mr. Johnson, we're showing that you owe a late fee for ANAL QUEENS 4."

SCORING

If your man scored 1–5, he doesn't have the balls to store porn in the house. If he could, he'd throw away all the books and stock the library with porn; but he's too afraid, so he resigns himself to renting porn when you go away or when he's away on business. Do this test again in a couple of years.

If your man scored 5–10, while not a certified porn king, he is definitely harboring a small stash somewhere in the house. If you care about finding it for your own "research" purposes, by all means do so. Or just confront him, and force him to open all of the things we listed above. If he's got a porn stash, he'll never do it.

If your man scored 10–20, check your man's ID, because his name may in fact be Larry Flynt. If he isn't Larry, he's running a close second. A chronic masturbator and purveyor of porn, your man has seen almost all of the new releases and can list porn movies and stars by name on cue. He spends at least $30–$50 per week renting porn, and actually knows what movies are coming out next month and can't wait to get his hands on them (then himself). At least make sure your man washes his hands a lot, because right after the average Joe is done with a video, he touches it and puts it back in the box. . . .

If your man scored over 20, your man doesn't have any porn in the house, *it's in his office!*

Meditation for the Day

"When I accuse (YOUR MAN'S NAME) of something and he denies it vehemently, chances are, just like O.J., he's absolutely 100% guilty."

20

HOW TO DETERMINE IF YOUR MAN *SECRETLY* WANTS A *THREESOME* WITH ANOTHER WOMAN

The first thing any SMITH AND DOE–educated woman needs to know is the following:

AS LONG AS HE THINKS IT WILL NOT DESTROY THE RELATION-SHIP (AND, OFTEN, EVEN IF HE DOES) EVERY MAN WANTS A THREESOME WITH AN ATTRACTIVE WOMAN AND YOU
(or anyone else, for that matter!).

Knowing this, realize that any man who claims to not want a threesome is most likely hiding a past strewn with threesomes. This way he figures you'll think, "Wow, he doesn't even want a threesome. What a sexually introverted guy. He would never cheat on me." Meanwhile, the guy has already probably had a threesome with the same girl you've got your eye on—except with someone else as the third!

Whether you are repulsed by or enamored with the idea of a threesome, understanding your man's position regarding it will empower you greatly in understanding the likelihood that he will stray. Because if your man wants a threesome badly, and you have no interest, and he's in a foreign country without you and has the opportunity to have a threesome, you're SOL ("Shit Out of Luck," in layman's terms).

THE FORMULA

$$PT = P + F + W + K \times PH \div PF$$

THE VARIABLES

P (Porn): The type of porn your man watches is a rare glimpse into the dark inner reaches of his sexual mind, since a man will rent porn that satisfies his needs. So if he feels like "having sex" with a redhead with a huge rack tonight instead of you, he'll rent a movie that has one of those in it. If he feels like gangbanging a short brunette with one leg, he'll rent one of those. You won't have any idea that there is any type of premeditation involved, but trust us, *there was always a reason behind every porn your man has ever rented*. Whether it be a type of sex or a certain face smiling at him from the box cover, there's a reason, and it's up to you to figure out what that reason is. Having said that, if your man rents porn that involves multiple partners OR, even worse, involves women only (girl-on-girl), then he is much more likely to be secretly wanting a threesome. Enter a number for this variable from **1–10, 1** being the standard, heterosexual, one-on-one porn, and **10** being an all-girl gangbang.

F (Friends): Does your man ever say how pretty one of your friends is and how much he'd like to "set her up" with a great guy friend of his? Well, you just met the enemy: Your man would love nothing more than for you to go to the hospital for a few days (nothing terminal) so he can have sex with that particular friend. Even better, he'd give two toes to have a threesome with you and her together. So, enter a **1, 2, or 3** in this box: a **1** if your man has never indicated such interest in a friend, a **2** if he has, and a **3** if he's brought it up more than once.

W (Watching): Is your man a particularly visual guy sexually? Does he like to watch you masturbate, or watch an excessive amount of porn? Does he always need to have the lights on, and/or like to be able to see your face during oral sex? While there's nothing wrong with being visually oriented, such a man is far more likely to want a threesome due to its highly visual nature. So put a **zero** if your man isn't, a **1** if he is very visual.

K (Knowledge): Once your man knows how you feel about a certain sexual topic, he will treat any discussion of it like a guy with palsy walking through a minefield: very carefully. *If you have indicated to your man that you are not interested in a threesome, he will never indicate his interest in it, ever, and you have just condemned yourself to a life devoid of the knowledge that your man is having threesomes behind your back with prostitutes.* Seem harsh? **SMITH AND DOE** have always said that if your man has an interest in something sexually and you aren't interested in giving it to him, he will get it, first mentally through masturbation then physically with another woman. So enter a **1–10** here: **1** if your man thinks you want a threesome, **10** if you've said you don't; if there's an in-between, use your best judgment.

PH (Past History): If your man's past is strewn with one-nighters, he has proven an insatiable craving for what **SMITH AND DOE** call *profound newness.* Your man needs something new all the time; it's not his fault, he just gets bored.

So if your man has had a lot of one-nighters in his past, regardless of what he tells you he feels now ("I've changed, that was the past!" Yeah, yeah, whatever!), put a **10** in for this variable. If your man had a few but not many, a **5**, and if your man was (and you've confirmed this secondhand, not just from him) a vestal virgin throughout most of his youth, a **1**. **IMPORTANT NOTE:** A man who has few sexual encounters not by choice but by virtue of being unattractive should get a **10** for this variable, *because people who had few sexual encounters because of physical or social problems during their youth that made them unattractive to the opposite sex spend the rest of their lives trying to catch up!*

PL (Pleased Factor): If you are finding yourself saying, "Is it almost over?" while pleasuring your man during oral sex, you've found that your man's Pleased Factor is high. This should not reflect poorly on you, it is simply the fact that your man has achieved a high threshold for satisfaction that requires additional stimulation. Men like this need stimuli, and what better stimuli than two girls instead of one? So if your man is hard to please, put a **1** here. If he's easy, put a **5**.

SCORING

If your man scored under 25, he has no interest in having a threesome with another woman. He's also probably gay and is desperately searching for some helmet to chow at gay bars every time he's lucky enough to go away on a business trip.

If your man scored from 25–100, your man would happily partake of a threesome, but you would have to do all the work. This means that you would have to get the girl, convince her to do it, and then tell your man what's happening and prod him to join the festivities. This is not a man who will be proactive, nor will he ever act proactive, even if deep inside he's dancing a jig.

If your man scored from 100–150, he wants a threesome and will never tell you he wants it. This is a man who is harboring wanton sexual desires that he feels might shock you and/or make you repulsed by him forever. To confirm our analysis, simply bring up the topic and say that you were thinking about doing it. While he would never jump up and celebrate, he will nonchalantly acquiesce as if it was a favor for you. The moment you leave the room, he will call all of his friends and tell them the great news. He'll also probably cancel the two hos he had scheduled to meet him during his next trip to Vegas.

If your man scored over 150, he wants threesomes, all right, but he will never tell you and he will never admit to wanting them, even if you ask for them. He may even go so far as to make you feel like a ho for suggesting it. THIS MAN IS DANGEROUS, because he doesn't trust you enough to show you a small piece of a dark side that would make the emperor in Star Wars look like a guy with no skeletons in his closet. You need to go to RED ALERT, read **SMITH AND DOE**'s first book—WHAT MEN DON'T WANT WOMEN TO KNOW—immediately, and prepare yourself for a life of mistrust, cheating with hos, and bold-faced lies.

Meditation for the Day

"When it comes to my man, I will only trust what I know firsthand—that which I've seen with my very own eyes. I will never mistake trust for truth."

21

HOW TO DETERMINE WHETHER OR NOT YOUR MAN HAS **PROBLEMS** *WITH YOUR* **APPEARANCE**

Yes. Well that's the simple answer, because he does. Have a problem or two, that is. But how can you really, definitively tell that your man isn't satisfied with your body and/or the way you dress?

Einstein couldn't create a formula to pinpoint your man's precise problems, but we can figure out the *level of discontent* your man is feeling. Does he secretly wish your hair were longer? That's no big deal. Does he secretly wish your body had an entirely different shape and size? That's a bigger deal.

THE FORMULA

$$CN = C + T + L + S + M \times WT \div SP$$

Note: CN = Contentedness

THE VARIABLES

C (Clothes): If your man has a problem with the way you dress, it's the least of your worries: It's an easy one to change. If your man has repeatedly told you that he's unhappy with the way you dress, don't ignore him. Appreciate his concerns and at least try to achieve a happy medium. But before you do that, put a **1** here if he has problems, a **zero** if he hasn't.

T (Tushy): A man who has conveyed unhappiness about the size of your butt is a man who has reached the end of his rope (every man knows how sensitive women are to the size of their butts, so conveying dissatisfaction is that much more dramatic). And we know "fixing it" isn't the easiest thing in the world. So if you have the problem of a large caboose attached to your backside and he's made a point to mention it, put a **1** here, a **zero** if not.

L (Legs): Put a **1** here if your man has complained in any way about your legs, a **zero** if he hasn't.

S (Skin): A man who references a zit or two you might have is a man who is secretly disgusted by it. Put a **1** here if he's mentioned it, a **zero** if he hasn't.

M (Magazines): If your man frequently looks through your Victoria's Secret catalog or any magazine full of beautiful women IN FRONT OF YOU, he is covertly sending a signal: GET IN SHAPE OR GET OUT. He's telling you, "Here's your competition, sitting right in the palm of my hands, and if you don't shape up you're going to be shipping out." Put a **1** here if he's looking at the mags, a **zero** if he isn't.

WT (What He's Told You): Unquestionably the most important variable in this equation. *What your man has actually told you is only a small fraction of what he really thinks and feels.* So you can rest assured that if he's vocalized one, some, or many of his concerns, the truth is much worse. So on a scale of **1–10, 1** being a man who's never mentioned any problems and **10** being a man who's always badgering you to change this or change that, plug in the number.

SP (Suspicion): No formula will work when the data's wrong, so we need to get an idea of how suspicious you are of your man's honesty. Maybe he hasn't ever mentioned a problem with your appearance, but do you really believe him? Is he too nice to say anything? Or is he too disgusted to even broach the subject?

If you believe that your man is honest and would tell you the truth about your appearance, plug a **1** in here. If you think your man may not have told you everything, but you can't be entirely sure, plug a **0.75** here. And if you think your man is a lying sack of shit who tells you you look great when he really thinks you look like the half-breed mongrel daughter of the Elephant Man, plug in a **0.5.**

SCORING

If your man scored under 10, he is very happy with your appearance, and if he has problems he's keeping them well-kept secrets.

If your man scored between 10–25, he thinks you could stand to make a few changes. And while no one's asking you to go out and get a nose and boob job, it can't hurt to acquiesce to a couple of his needs, just to be a team player.

If your man scored between 25–50, you are skating on thin ice, at least in his eyes. You may need to hit the gym, plastic surgeon, and dermatologist all at the same time. Talk to him, find out his problems (but if he got this score you probably know his problems already), and try your best to deal with them. If there's nothing you can do or his requests are unreasonable, give him the boot and hit the local hair club for men to find yourself a new one.

If your man scored over 50, he thinks you are physically repugnant. Maybe he's staying with you because you're very wealthy, or because he needs something else you've got. Maybe you're his best friend and he's banging the receptionist at work, so he's got all his bases covered. Our advice is to either move to Pakistan where you can keep your face covered the whole time or try to find someone who will find you attractive, like Stevie Wonder.

Meditation for the Day

"The second (YOUR MAN'S NAME) *has his orgasm, where I am becomes the last place on earth he wants to be."*

22

HOW TO DETERMINE **WHAT YOU CAN DO** *TO MAKE YOUR MAN CARE MORE ABOUT* **YOUR ORGASMS**

As if there hasn't been enough written about your orgasms. How *earth-shattering* are they, how *long* do they go on, how *many* of them do you have? Are you sick of the word *"multiple"* yet? Are you tired of *reading* about "multiple orgasms" but never *having* them?

First off, whatever your problem (assuming you have one, and our research shows that 83.8% of women do), it lies with you but it's not you—it's the person lying next to you—your man.

Sexual science has demonstrated that most men go along blithely assuming they're fantastic lovers, totally unaware of how truly insignificant and unsatisfying their feeble attempts at lovemaking are. They act like the greatest thing you can ever do for them is to *let them* come in your mouth, and the greatest thing they can do for you is to *come* in your mouth. Have they never seen a woman's magazine? Are they totally ignorant of the *female orgasm?*

The answer is **ATTITUDE.** The value your man places on

your sexual fulfillment is the **ATTITUDE** he has toward *your sexual pleasure.* It all stems from his *underlying motivation.* Is his motivation simply to "unload"? To do whatever it takes to have his orgasm? In his mind, are you a *partner* for sex or a *tool* for unloading? This is what we mean by his **ATTITUDE.** You must be aware of this underlying motivation, or **ATTITUDE,** in order to teach him that making love is *as much about you as it is about him.*

In pursuit of this goal, we are therefore providing a formula by which you can determine his sexual **ATTITUDE** toward you. Armed with the results of this equation you can proceed to go about his training more efficiently and with greater (or should we say *"multiple"*) results.

THE FORMULA

$$A = (HO - YO) \times (HNS - YNS)$$

Stated in layman's terms, this means *the difference between the number of orgasms each of you have per week* multiplied by *the difference between the number of times each of you want to have sex per week* equals his ATTITUDE toward your orgasms. How does it work? Read on.

THE VARIABLES

(HO) His Orgasms per week.

My man has approximately ____ orgasms per week (with me).
1 or less **(11 points)**
2 **(12 points)**

3 (**13 points**)

4 (**14 points**)

5 (**15 points**)

6 or more (**20 points**)

(YO) Your Orgasms per week.

I have approximately ___ orgasms per week (with him).

1 or less (**1 point**)

2 (**2 points**)

3 (**4 points**)

4 (**5 points**)

6 or more (**10 points**)

(YSN) Your Sexual Needs per week.

I need to have sex approximately ___ times per week (with him).

1 or less (**11 points**)

2 (**12 points**)

3 (**13 points**)

4 (**14 points**)

5 (**15 points**)

6 or more (**20 points**)

(HSN) His Sexual Needs per week.

He needs to have sex approximately ___ times per week (with me).

1 or less (**1 point**)

2 (**2 points**)

3 (**3 points**)

4 (**4 points**)

5 (5 points)

6 or more (10 points)

SCORING
From *your* point of view

The *worst* score he can get is 361, which means he has more orgasms than you; therefore, he needs to have sex less often than you (thereby giving *you* even fewer orgasms).

The *best* score he can get is 1, which means he has fewer orgasms than you; therefore, he needs to have sex more than you (thereby giving you *even more* orgasms!).

Note: If you discover a a man who scores 1, bring him immediately to the Smithsonian Museum—
he's the only one (1) ever found!

WHAT YOU CAN DO

If he scored 300–361, he's an irredeemable megalomaniac who assumes the word *"pleasure"* means *"Me first."* The only thing you can do with a case like this is come up with a hard dollar amount in your mind—which you will eventually take out of his bank account or his hide—for each time he doesn't give you the same pleasure he got from you.

If he scored 250–300, it's more like he's hopelessly lost and needs a road map. Borrow a medical poster of female sexual organs from your gynecologist's office, hang it over your bed, and get yourself a laser pointer. As your man is becoming excited, call his attention to the poster and indicate with the pointer exactly where he needs to pay attention in order for you to pay attention to him. If he's Mr. Right he'll be grateful for the advice. If he's Mr. Wrong he'll squeal like a stuck pig. In any case, he won't resent you so much for making *him* unload *you* before *you* unload *him* if you make it seem like a macho game—*he* is "driving" (along your erotic zones) and must reach his "destination" (your orgasm) to "save the world." Only after he "saves the world" will you rock his.

If he scored 200–250, he's more salvageable than the last guy, but not much. The good news is, he's probably conscious that women want orgasms. The bad news, his consciousness deserts him during sex. The trick is to snap him out of it before his climax. A glass of cold water, a slap on the back of his head, a baring of teeth during oral sex . . . be creative. He'll get the message.

If he scored 100–200, he's a little better than average. This man is well intentioned and capable of producing the *multiple* if you train him properly.

If he scored 1–100, he's a keeper. Heed the old adage: "If it ain't broke, don't fix it."

☺

Meditation for the Day

"If, without my asking, (YOUR MAN'S NAME) tells me about a sexual need, I will take it very seriously, for he will rarely tell me twice. If he doesn't get what he asks for from me, he will certainly get it elsewhere."

GAUGING YOUR MAN'S MADONNA-WHORE COMPLEX

Whether you are aware of it or not, your man's sexual openness is impacted to a stultifying degree by the **Madonna-Whore Complex** (**MWC**). This is a sexual state of being in which the male confuses his female sex partner with his mother (but not, fortunately, the converse). *For some reason still undetermined, this condition is less prominent among atheists than in religious cults such as Jews and Catholics. (And now that we're at it, why do we capitalize "Jews" and "Catholics" but not **"atheists"**? This will be explained in **SMITH AND DOE**'s next bombshell, **"The Big Book of Bigotry."**)*

When a man is in an ongoing relationship with a woman, he begins to subconsciously identify that woman with his mother, the most influential of all his previous heterosexual relationships. The longer the relationship lasts, the more the boundaries of his initial lust appear to contract during sex, becoming narrower and narrower until he subconsciously merges her in his mind with . . . *his mother.*

The key word here is **subconsciously**. If he *knew* what he was doing, he would throw up on the spot.

The proof of this theory is in the pudding. On a first date, when there is no ***relationship*** per se, if you go to bed with him he performs like a wanton sex animal *(which you want)*. But with each little ratcheting up and deepening of the relationship, his subconscious will identify little things about you with similar little things about his mother *(**the Madonna**)*. The more he interacts with you, the more you resemble his mother.

Now this is not all bad. Hopefully, he treats his mother with ***respect and consideration***, and this is certainly how you wish to be treated. But sexually, there's a problem. He begins to become inhibited. When you've become *more* than just a lover—when you've become part lover/part mother—he begins to treat you ***sexually*** as if you *were* his mother—with *too much* respect and consideration. The wild abandon, the crazy explorations, the daring positions begin to evaporate. There are things he would never do with his mother that he would do with, say, a prostitute. The reason he would not do them is because he would not want to risk the moral disapproval of his mother.

For instance, he would never ask his *mother* to pee on him, even if that is what he wants from a woman more than anything else. It's immoral. But a prostitute, with whom he has *no relationship*, well, that's another story. (Asking a prostitute to pee on him is about *money* and steaming hot urine, not morals.)

Basically, the more he confuses you with his mother, the less likely he is to ask you to pee on him. Now, we're **not** saying you want to pee on him. But you *are* his lover, and he should be able to ask his lover to do anything. Even if his lover refuses, communication has been established where there was none before.

When a man is in the grasp of the **Madonna-Whore Complex**, he is unable to fully communicate his sexual desires. Of course, *peeing* is an extreme desire. But *for him*, anything beyond the "missionary" position constitutes going beyond the bounds of **the Madonna's** moral approval. *(After all, it was **the Madonna** who toilet-trained him in the first place.)* For instance, if he wants to approach you in the rear, he may not be able to tell you that because of the **MWC**. He is intimidated by having to say such a thing to **the Madonna** part of you.

The **MWC** is one of the greatest problems in sexual relationships. Because it is so humiliating to men, **it is never discussed**. And if you try to bring it up, he'd rather die than admit the nasty things he would like to do. And even if he did admit them, he would never do those things *with you* because he has already identified you with his mother.

Catch-22? Not necessarily.

There is hope, but you need to break through his **MWC**, shatter the little identifications he has made between you and Mom, and get him to open up about his sexual desires, thereby giving you the rare opportunity to see how deeply embedded he is in the **MWC**. Our formula will give you a good idea of how much he has succumbed to the complex and provide suggestions for coping with his level of debilitation.

THE FORMULA

$$100\% - TT\% - SC\% - ATM\% = MWC$$

Note: **MCW = Degree to which his sexuality with you is negatively affected by the Madonna-Whore Complex**

THE VARIABLES

(TT) Time Together. This refers to the length of time you have had an *ongoing* relationship with your man, including the time (if any) before you began having sex with him. This begins to point the way to how much his picture of you has merged with his picture of Mom.

My man and I have had an
ongoing relationship for . . .
1 year or less (**30%**)
1–2 years (**20%**)
2–3 years (**15%**)
3–4 years (**10%**)
4–5 years (**8%**)
5–10 years (**4%**)
more than 10 years (**2%**)

(SC) Sexual Creativity. How creative is he? How often does he come up with something new to try? How willing is he to try something *you* come up with? Has he ever made a *bizarre* request? Has he ever wanted to watch *bizarre* sex videos with you? This is a general gauge of his degree of sexual inhibition.

My man follows the same sexual script . . .
All the time (**2%**)
Most of the time (**10%**)
Some of the time (**15%**)
Hardly ever (**25%**)
Never (**32%**)

(ATM) Attachment to Mom. This is a judgment call based on *your own observations*. Despite the proverbial "Jewish mother" type, no particular group of moms has a monopoly on apron strings. Most mothers retain *some* degree of influence over their sons. From the choices below, select the one that *best describes your assessment* of your man's attachment to his mom.

In my opinion, **my man's mother . . .**
Has a normal and reasonable relationship with him **(34%)**
Is his psychological Siamese twin **(30%)**
Is like the hall monitor to my man's naughty student **(20%)**
Usually controls him like a dog on a leash **(10%)**
Has him totally by the balls and can never be pried loose
(0%)

SCORING

100% − TT% − SC% − ATM% = MWC

The *best* he can get is 14%—his sexuality
***with you* is negatively affected only 14% by the**
Madonna-Whore Complex
[100% − 14% − 32% − 40% = 14%]

The *worst* he can get is 96%—his sexuality
***with you* is negatively affected 96% by the**
Madonna-Whore Complex
[100% − 2% − 2% − 0% = 96%]

**If he scored 14%–24%: GOOD NEWS: No other woman
is urinating on your guy.** BETTER NEWS: It won't be long
before he asks you to try it *(an encouraging sign of his
MWC-free sexuality.)* **SMITH AND DOE** SUGGEST: Rubber
sheets and plenty of towels.

**If he scored 25%–50%: GOOD NEWS: You're not fully
merged with his mother. BAD NEWS: You haven't been
with him long enough to complete the process. SMITH
AND DOE** SUGGEST: Get him to wear your clothing. Or give
you a spanking. Or send *you* to bed without dinner. Beg,
plead, implore on your hands and knees if you have to, but

get him to do things to merge *himself* with his mother instead of merging *you* with her.

If he scored 50%–75%: BAD NEWS: He'll start kidding around and trying to be cool by calling you "Mama"— like, "Get down, Mama," or "You my funky Mama." WORSE NEWS: He means it. SMITH AND DOE SUGGEST: Emergency action—this could backfire but you have no choice. Dress up in his mother's clothes and wear his mother's perfume and nag him mercilessly until he either begins to hate her or turns gay.

If he scored 75%–90%: GOOD NEWS: NONE. SMITH AND DOE SUGGEST: Tell him he can stick his mother up his ass, pleasure yourself, and move on.

IN CONCLUSION: A WORD IN OUR OWN DEFENSE

We are aware of the vilification that will accrue to us as a result of publishing this book. Feminist pundits, high-brow males, and "serious" reviewers will look down their shiny clean noses at the truths we have dared to reveal and vent hailstorms of pompous outrage in their eagerness to drown out our voices.

And yet, on your behalf, dear lover of truth, we will not surrender.

On your behalf we will not be intimidated.

SMITH AND DOE stand behind everything we have written.

To those revolted by the mention of smelly vaginas we say, *"Cleanse thyself!"*

To those horrified by craven cash value applied to sexual worth we say, *"If you don't like it, get a real job!"*

To those sickened by "normal" men wearing lipstick we say, *"If you can't stand the flaming mo, get him out of your kitchen!"*

We realize the hostile reactions of these so-called "critics" are a classic example of killing the messenger simply because of the message—and yet we are determined to stand by our principles, to risk everything for the money.

So if something you've learned about someone you know makes you feel like doing something terrible to **SMITH AND DOE,** count to ten and remember one indisputable fact—*the truth always hurts.*